PreMed

Who Makes It
and Why

MARY ANN MAGUIRE

Foreword by David Mechanic

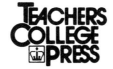

TEACHERS
COLLEGE
PRESS

Teachers College, Columbia University
New York and London

Published by Teachers College Press, 1234 Amsterdam Avenue, New York, NY 10027

Library of Congress Cataloging-in-Publication Data

Maguire, Mary Ann 1946–
    PreMed : who makes it and why / Mary Ann Maguire.
    p.   cm. — (Sociology of education series)
  Includes bibliographical references and index.
  ISBN 0-8077-3833-6 (cloth : alk. paper)
  ISBN 0-8077-3832-8 (pbk. : alk. paper)
    1. Premedical education—United States—Longitudinal studies.   I.
Title. II. Series.
  R838 .M34 1999
  610'.71'173—dc21   98-48715

ISBN 0-8077-3832-8 (paper)
ISBN 0-8077-3833-6 (cloth)

Printed on acid-free paper

Manufactured in the United States of America

06   05   04   03   02   01   00   99   8   7   6   5   4   3   2   1

CONTENTS

FOREWORD

Social selection shapes almost every aspect of living, from mating and child-bearing to the choice of occupation or profession. Some life choices are almost incidental, a product of drift and coincidence. Others require early anticipation, planning, preparation, extensive effort, and persistence. Few occupations require as much prior thought and persistence as a career in medicine, but once admitted to medical school, the probability is exceedingly high that the student will one day be a physician. So while there are many years of hard work and commitment required, the crucial challenge is getting through the door. In a readable style, Mary Ann Maguire describes how a group of undergraduates made their way through a premed curriculum and helps us understand why some reached their goal of medical school admission and others did not.

Planning to become a doctor for most students begins early. Mary Ann Maguire finds that a majority of the students she followed who were accepted to medical school had aspired to become doctors before high school. Making such an early choice sets the stage for developing the study habits needed and for taking the right courses in preparation for the challenges of the college premed curriculum. Premed students need not be geniuses, but they require the ability and discipline to perform reasonably well in the required science and math courses, to prepare for the MCAT, and to proceed on the increasingly demanding journey of medical school and residency.

The premed curriculum, along with earlier schooling experiences, help build the study habits and coping strategies that are later called on as academic demands increase in medical school. Medical faculty may bemoan the memorizing and other coping strategies students adopt to "make the grade," but they inevitably contribute to it by the impossible challenges they pose. This may not be as irrational as some have suggested because the profession of doctoring itself involves uncertainties and an incomplete grasp of all the pertinent information available. Students learn to be good doctors by understanding their limitations, by taking intelligent shortcuts and avoiding imprudent ones, and understanding the importance of learning how to continue to learn.

As Mary Ann Maguire indicates, there may be many considerations in admission to medical school, but mastery of the requisite science and math courses and good performance on the MCAT are key factors. No one should doubt that such basic preparation is important in a profession so greatly dependent on a fast-moving scientific frontier, although one often hears complaints about the irrelevance of these studies. However, what is less clear is how such studies are properly combined with the range of other skills in behavioral science, epidemiology, informatics, clinical decision-making, and other subject matter increasingly important for the future practice of medicine. How well a student does in math and science courses and on the MCAT predicts successful performance in the preclinical years in medical school, but it is much less clear that it predicts who will be outstanding physicians.

This study by Mary Ann Maguire makes a useful contribution by focusing on the premed years, whereas other authors have focused on medical school education. More has been written on medical education than the education of members of any other profession. Many have pondered how to instill the skills and strengths of character to facilitate judgment and caring as well as scientific acuity. Some worry that the focus on basic science and academic competitiveness select candidates who would lack the ideal temperament to care deeply for patients in their care. Others are concerned that the prestige and relatively high financial rewards of medicine select aspirants for the wrong reasons. These debates will, no doubt, go on. The fact remains that the profession of medicine has been persistently successful in attracting candidates of talent who are strongly motivated to contribute usefully to society. Maguire's examination of the premed students' motivation portrays their high ideals. If some doctors are corrupted along the way, the reasons are often more connected to the incentives and constraints in which their work is embedded than in initial aspirations.

As Mary Ann Maguire notes in her book, medical work is being transformed, and student physicians now face new uncertainties and concerns. Future doctors will work more frequently in highly organized settings, have less personal autonomy, and face more social and economic demands. They will work more frequently in groups and with other professionals, in both a cooperative yet also competitive fashion. There is little doubt, however, that a good grasp of science, increasingly broader in scope, will remain intrinsic to the task and to future advances in health. But the debate on how to properly socialize the physician for this future will continue.

—*David Mechanic*
Institute for Health,
Health Care Policy,
and Aging Research
Rutgers University

PREFACE

Before I had thought about this study, I had occasion to speak one-on-one with several students in their first year of college and in their first semester of a premed program. Each of them was giving some thought to withdrawing from general chemistry, the first of the required premed courses. They found the course difficult, and other students seemed to be far better prepared than they were. These other students were thought to have attended better high schools, to have had better teachers, or to have completed 2 years of chemistry while still in high school. I did not accept the students' rationale at face value.

I was surprised that students who had identified themselves as premed on entering college were so quickly discouraged from pursuing their goal. Although some might attempt the course again, most probably would not. The two-semester chemistry course sequence would not begin again until the fall semester, so those students who planned to take it up again would delay their premed progress by a full year. While I knew that many students found the curriculum difficult, I knew, too, that a premed course of study anywhere has this reputation. Furthermore, the contents of this curriculum have not changed in decades and by now should be well known. Why would students beginning college in a premed program change their plans so quickly? To address this question, I conducted a few informal interviews with students, but the results did not satisfy my curiosity.

I spoke with the chair of a university chemistry department and asked why students who had done well enough in high school chemistry could not necessarily expect to continue doing well in college-level chemistry. He responded that many high school courses are less quantitative and more descriptive than those taught in college; consequently, grades earned in the high school course are poor predictors of success in the college course. He also told me, contrary to the opinion of the first-year students with whom I had spoken, that relatively few students taking general chemistry in college had completed 2 years of the subject in high school. Students who do well, he said, are those with good quantitative backgrounds or at least a willingness to tackle quantitative material. What advice could he give to those students who wished to do well? "Do all of the problems at the end of each chapter in the textbook." As his response did not convince me, I was certain that it would not persuade first-year premed students who doubted that they could succeed.

Soon thereafter I had occasion to talk with a college senior majoring in chemistry. She was doing well in the subject. I asked if she had had a good high school course. "No," she said. A good teacher? "Not especially." There were no laboratory facilities for student use at her small rural school, and the lab portion of their course was limited to occasional demonstrations by the teacher. Yet she earned an A in both of her first two semesters of college chemistry. I asked how she had done it. "I did all of the problems at the end of the chapters," was her response. I was beginning to catch on. Some current premed students also recognized the wisdom in this advice: "The key to it all is doing all the problems at the end of the chapter. I didn't do this in general chemistry," one premed student said. The consequence of not doing problems is less familiarity with the applications of theories and methods and less of the discipline that is built from attempting the problems whether you want to or not. Yet just doing the problems does not yield admission to medical school. The 4-year progression through a premed program is far more complex than that simple prescription would suggest.

I have never been a premed student (but I did take two semesters of college chemistry), nor have I ever thought about medicine as a career for myself. My interest in undertaking research on students in a premedicine program was to make sense of something I did not understand, to know more about the significant decisions these young men and women were making—why some students complete that demanding program and others do not. Are the persistent better prepared? Or just more highly motivated? Or differently motivated? Or receiving more support from family and friends? I learned that many students who begin as premeds in their first year of college are not well informed about what will be expected of them over the next several years. While some premeds retain the dream of being a doctor, they do not complete the program after performing poorly in required courses. Some who did well in high school by exerting little effort find college, and especially the premed curriculum, to be far more difficult, and they are unwilling or unable to devote the effort necessary to succeed. For others it is the social life and other enjoyment foregone that is too great a cost to bear while they are young and in college. Some premeds lose interest or discover new interests and future directions that they regard as more appealing. For some of them, this is the shedding of medicine, their parents' dream for them, in favor of their own dream.

In attempting to answer the question of persistence, I took a long view and designed the study reported here. I became acquainted with research by Robert Fiorentine and others that compared male and female premed students' persistence in premed programs. The focus of that research was on the support that these students received from others and on the different experiences of men and women premeds. My own initial interest, and one that continued throughout the study, was in the role played by interest in and mastery of science in the persistence of men and women in premed. I chose a selective private university for the study, on the assumption that a sufficient number of students at that institution would persist in premed and would gain acceptance to a medical school. What began as an idle question about some puzzling student behavior became a lengthy research project for me as I followed two cohorts of self-declared premed students through their college years.

In 1989 I invited all first-year liberal arts (not engineering) students in general chemistry to join the study if they were premed. I repeated the same invitation to first-year students in 1990. The project began with 153 participants, 87 women and 66 men; students who left the premed program were no longer participants in the study. In their last year of college, 34 women and 18 men were still in the study. Participants gave permission to extract from their college files information on their backgrounds, high school experiences, and grades. The rest of the data were collected in three interviews, using quantitative and also qualitative items. While the data were collected from students in a single institution, the premed curriculum and much about the premed experience is similar across institutions. A longitudinal study such as this one provides the opportunity to follow individuals as they changed their behaviors, priorities, opinions, and aspirations over time. This project was to a degree exploratory; a wide range of issues was covered in the interviews in an attempt to try to understand what these students were going through. The study reported here began before the start of the Clinton presidency, just before the reform of the national health care system became a high priority. As the study progressed through 5 years, there was additional anxiety for premed students, who wondered whether the structure of medicine would change in ways that would exclude them.

While this book is not intended to be a how-to manual for medical school acceptance, there is much for aspiring and current premeds to learn from some of their recent predecessors. It is possible to state in a concise way what is required to gain acceptance to medical school—academic achievement in science as well as overall, a demonstrated commitment to medicine, interpersonal skills, and involvement in some extracurricular activities. Yet the path in pursuit of the goal is not clearly defined. There are numerous opportunities for decision and action throughout this lengthy process of pursuing a medical career. There also are many and various interpretations of these choice situations and reactions to them made by individuals facing them. The voices of some premed students will be heard throughout this book, giving their personal perspectives on these 4 years. Literature on the profession of medicine, on the occupational choice process, and on gender and science provided a context for interpreting the experience of these premeds.

The premeds in the study, especially those who continued in their pursuit of admission to medical school, participated with great interest. For most of these students, who combined long hours in classes and laboratories with part-time employment, community service, and their other interests and relationships, college was a time of stress, with little time for fun. One student told me that he wished he had some time that wasn't structured, time for "hanging out" with friends, but he had no such time. This book should help current and future premed students, their friends, families, teachers, and counselors, as well as students of education and occupation, understand and appreciate the experience of these doctor hopefuls.

ACKNOWLEDGMENTS

I am grateful for the assistance of many colleagues, family members, and friends in the implementation of this study and in the writing of this book. To the men and women whose participation throughout 4 years of data collection made the book possible, I am most grateful. My thanks go, too, to those medical school faculty and staff whom I interviewed and to Susan Seguin at the Association of American Medical Colleges. Ann Die, William Cooper, Jeanie Watson, and Valerie Greenberg provided support at key stages of this project. I am grateful to Julie Hauber, Kerri MacDonald, Beth Willinger, and Beth Poe for their assistance and support, and to Paula Carter for interviewing students, Jennifer Sweet for coding data, and Patricia Kasari and especially Rachel Jones for data analysis. The Newcomb Foundation provided funds for interviewing, coding, and early data analysis. The reference and interlibrary loan staffs of the Howard Tilton Library at Tulane University were helpful in locating reference materials. Thanks go to Jim March, who introduced me to the study of choice, to Sandy Dornbusch for assistance with the book at an early stage, to the anonymous reviewers who read earlier drafts of the manuscript, and to editors Susan Liddicoat and Gary Natriello.

I am grateful for the moral support of my parents, John and Mary Maguire, throughout my life. Finally, a very special thanks to my patient and understanding husband, Rockwell Livingston, to whom this book is dedicated.

FROM THE SERIES EDITOR

By following a cohort of college students through their premedical studies, this volume demonstrates the utility of sociological analyses of educational processes for others involved or soon to be involved in similar processes. There is much in this study to inform other students contemplating a career in medicine to guide them through their undergraduate programs. Both students and their parents will appreciate the insights gained through a careful examination of the experiences of the men and women followed in this study, both those who eventually enrolled in medical school and those who did not.

This study also offers sociologists of education a sound model for the examination of an important part of the schooling career. Although the data were gathered from undergraduate premedical students, by carefully inquiring about the high school and earlier childhood experiences of these students and by following some of them for a period of time after they completed their undergraduate degrees, the study offers an extended longitudinal view of students making the transition from high school to college and then onto professional school. The study combines quantitative summaries with case reports on individual students to document and illustrate the major elements in the premedical curriculum and their impact on these highly able students.

Chapter 1

INTRODUCTION

"Premed is very demanding; you have to be dedicated and really want it."*

This book is about young men and women who aspire to be doctors—how they arrived at college with this aspiration (or dream), how their goals were strengthened or changed in college, why many of them still are interested in medicine when they leave college, and why some are not. Their story is one of hard work and tenacity by young adults, virtually all of whom want to make the world a better place. Yet good intentions and effort are not enough, as there is an excess of applicants for spaces in the next medical school class. That structure of opportunity, as well as a set of demanding required courses, produces competition, anxiety, and disappointment, as well as the joy that accompanies acceptance. While medicine accepts applications from rich and poor, persons from all racial and ethnic groups, older and younger (but mostly younger) men and women, what successful applicants have in common is superior performance in a college premed program.

Medicine, as the term is used in this book, refers to allopathic medicine, as opposed to osteopathic and homeopathic medicine. *Profession* refers to an occupation that entails higher education and advanced training, is built upon a body of theoretical knowledge, has its own code of ethics and a procedure for enforcing the code, and serves the public. Bullough (1966) noted the association between profession and religious vows: "a person who entered a profession did so, or at least attempted to give the impression that he did, with something other than the profit motive in mind" (p. 3). This use of the term *profession* is distinct from the way in which it is used in current advertising, where the term is used synonymously with *high quality*.

One survey of "the general public" asked respondents which of 10 professional occupations deserved the most respect. The most frequent response, at 30%, was clergy, with doctors at 28%. Five years later, "when

---

*Unless otherwise identified, all quotations are from the interviews with study participants.

I

respondents were asked which profession they would recommend to a son or daughter . . . medicine (24%) led all responses" ("What Americans Really Think About Lawyers," 1986, quoted in Moll, 1991, p. 7). Is there any reason, then, to ask why medicine as a profession is attractive to young men and women and, even earlier, to boys and girls? Apart from complaints about managed care and the *business* that medicine has become, individual doctors are respected—by their patients and in their communities. They do good for others, and they earn high incomes. For many individuals, their doctor is the most accomplished and successful person they know.

In spite of the high rewards, however, only 5% of first-year college students nationwide aspire to be doctors (Astin, 1990). Who wants to be a doctor, when the costs of time and money are factored in? And, among those who begin working toward the goal of medical school acceptance and eventually a medical practice, who still wants to be a doctor 4 years later and who gets the opportunity? This study of a sample of premed students explores those questions.

THE STUDY

The 153 students who participated in this study were enrolled in one highly selective university. Yet they were a heterogeneous group, spanning a wide range of family income, parental occupation, high school quality, and geographic region. They were Caucasian, African American, Asian American, Hispanic, and Native American. All of the study participants were college freshmen in 1989 or 1990, enrolled in a liberal arts and sciences program of study that included general chemistry, the first of the premed courses. Students who were in this course but were not premed were not included in the study. Virtually all were of traditional college age, 17 to 19 years, when they began college; more than half were women. Their high school cumulative grade-point averages (GPAs) in academic subjects ranged from 2.11 to 4.00, with a mean of 3.41. (Their high school grade-point averages had been recomputed by the admission's office to include only academic courses; this had the result of making the set of courses on which the GPA was computed more comparable across students.) Approximately 30% of the entering classes in 1989 and 1990 self-identified as premed, six times the rate among their peers nationwide who said they wanted to be doctors. Katchadourian and Boli (1994) noted about Stanford students a decade earlier:

> Over one-third of our entering class professed some interest in medicine, but only 13% became doctors. Many of the rest could not hack their way through

the premed jungle. Others who were equal to the task became disenchanted or developed other interests. (p. 63)

The premed students I studied were not different from their classmates as a whole in their level of performance in high school; over half of their cohort had graduated in the top 20% of their high school classes. They scored slightly higher than their classmates on the Scholastic Aptitude Test (SAT) or American College Testing Program (ACT). They averaged 572 on the verbal portion of the exams and 601 on the quantitative portion (642 and 601 when converted to the new, recentered SAT scale originating in 1996). ACT scores were converted to an SAT scale. Most of the premeds and their fellow students had completed a high school curriculum of 4 years of mathematics, science, and English, and 3 to 4 years of foreign language and of history/social science.

The study participants were asked for permission to retrieve from their college records information on their applications for admission and on their high school and college transcripts. The admission material contained information on the high school(s) attended; experiences while in high school, including extracurricular activities and employment; high school courses taken and grades earned; SAT/ACT scores; and family characteristics, including birth order, parents' education, and parents' occupations. The students had provided this information during the first part of their last year in high school and were doing so for *official* purposes, for college admission. Consequently, these data are less susceptible to the distortion that can affect survey responses to questions about past events. The further away respondents are from their experience, the more questionable is their undocumented recollection of these experiences and the contexts in which they occurred.

The remaining data were collected in three interviews, most of which I conducted, with the aid of some student assistants, at the close of the first, second, and fourth years of college. They covered academic, pre-professional, familial, extracurricular, and social issues. In a very real sense, this was a collaborative effort between me and the study participants, who provided insights in their responses that had not previously been apparent to me. If students transferred to another institution, they were not contacted for further interviews. If they left premed, a final interview was scheduled. If they did not respond to multiple requests to schedule an interview, they were not pursued further, although their data until that point, as well as course enrollments and grades earned, are included here. Consequently, even these students could still be classified as premed or not throughout their college years.

That the respondents did not feel constrained by the interviewer to answer questions in one way rather than another was illustrated by their willingness to provide negative evaluations of some of their experiences, including naming professors with whom they were dissatisfied. They were assured that their names would not be associated with their responses. The interviews were conducted privately and not tape-recorded, so their answers to questions reflect their true feelings to the best extent possible. One student went so far as to preface a comment with "I've never told this to anyone before." Because study participants were so interested in the subject at hand, most of them participated actively in the interviews. On a couple of occasions, individuals even expressed concern when they had not been contacted to schedule the next interview at a time when they thought interviews should be taking place; they feared the study had been discontinued.

PREMED PROFILE

Three-quarters of the premeds lived with two parents. In some cases a student lived with a parent and a stepparent, but the bonds within the family were sufficiently close for the student to characterize the family type as *two parent*. Most of the remaining students lived with one parent (nearly always their mother) while in high school, and a few lived with someone else, usually another relative. Nationally, the family profile of college students was similar, with 72% of students entering college in 1989 living in two-parent families (Astin, 1990). Fathers of our students were likely to have completed at least a bachelor's degree (69%); 41% had completed a graduate or professional degree. Nearly half (46%) of their mothers had completed at least a bachelor's degree and 16%, a graduate or professional degree. The national data on parents' education show a less well educated population of parents, with 42% of fathers and 32% of mothers of college freshmen with bachelor's degrees or more. Eighteen percent of fathers and 10% of mothers held graduate degrees (Astin, 1990).

Fathers of the premed students were most likely to be in managerial or professional occupations, including 13% who were physicians. Mothers, too, were more likely to be in managerial or professional occupations than in any other category, while 20% were homemakers and not employed outside the home. Family sizes ranged from one to eight children, with a mode of two. While it was somewhat more common to be the older or oldest child than to be the youngest or in the middle, there was substantial variation in the birth order of respondents. When asked to report their family's annual income, using five categories, the single *category* selected more than any other was $75,001–$100,000, although most families earned less. Family income of college freshmen nationally in 1989 showed that the category $25,000–$49,999 was the largest (Astin, 1990). While there was variation in the socioeconomic characteristics of this premed population, as a group they were better off than the population of college students as a whole.

INFLUENCES ON PERSISTENCE

Every career is a set of choices, including opportunities foregone or ignored, as well as those more conscious actions taken to reach goals. When the occupation is one requiring lengthy training and entailing intense competition just to access this training, the aspirants become acutely aware that they are always being tested. At each of a number of identifiable steps along the way, they are faced with a decision—to stay or to leave. The decision may not be freely taken, an expression of a preference, but instead may be a recognition that "I don't have what it takes." Medicine is such a career. Among those students who enter college as premeds, a majority will not complete the program, a smaller percentage will apply to at least one medical school, and a still smaller number will gain admission. A small fraction of the original group of interested men and women will progress on the way to becoming doctors. An additional form of uncertainty presents itself to individuals preparing for a career in medicine today—an uncertainty about how medicine will be practiced in the future, in the light of public discussions about restructuring the delivery of health care.

Four sets of factors, which I will examine throughout this book, impact on persistence toward the goal of becoming a doctor as early as childhood for some individuals and throughout college for all. The first is academic achievement and the effort that supports this achievement—courses taken, grades earned, time available, and effort applied. The second set of factors is the social: support from family and others on the positive side and competition from fellow students on the negative. Gender is the third factor, whose impact has changed in nature and degree over time with an increase in the number of women completing premed requirements and applying to medical schools. The fourth factor, attraction to medicine and its anticipated rewards, is measured first when the premeds are in college.

Academic Achievement

Academic achievement refers not only to grades in science courses but also to academic performance across subjects and to scores on standardized tests. Students who are not particularly interested in science but regard premed and medical school science courses as obstacles to be overcome en route to eventual clinical practice will be at a disadvantage. Likewise, students who have an interest in science but lack an aptitude for science and mathematics will have difficulty demonstrating the necessary competence.

The sort of effort that contributes to academic success includes studying—knowing what to study and how—and the commitment to a long-range goal, sticking with it month after month and year after year, even when progress toward the goal is slow or stalled. To the degree that individuals while still in high school have committed themselves to an activity or goal in the past, they have acquired behaviors that contribute to persistence. An example of such behavior includes taking advanced placement and honors courses, which have heavier workloads than other high school courses and in which mastery of material requires extra concentration and time. The habit of commitment can also be developed with consistent involvement in the same extracurricular activity throughout high school and by assuming leadership roles—becoming proficient on the violin or on the basketball court, or being elected president of the debate society. Students who learn to make these commitments while still in high school should have less difficulty making a commitment to a rigorous academic program in college.

Academic success is affected, too, by some contextual factors over which the individual has little or no control. Students do not control the quality of classroom instruction, the breadth of course offerings at their school, or the adequacy of their laboratory facilities. Nor can they always control the outside distractions that reduce the time available for concentrated study. Some students have more extensive household responsibilities, including the care of siblings or other family members. Others must put in time as needed at a family business.

Social Factors

Social factors include support from family and friends for the long-term goal of becoming a doctor and for the more immediate behavior required to reach the goal, including quiet time to study for difficult science courses. Social factors extend beyond support, however, to include competition—with other bright students in high schools or colleges, as well as nationwide. Support alone without academic achievement or perceived reward is not likely to keep a student in premed. Nor would we expect to find that individuals with high levels of achievement in science drop out because of a lack of support. Social support is more important during the high school years, when the young man or woman is making initial career-related decisions regarding course choices, college applications, and the allocation of attention across competing interests. College, in contrast, is a time for making choices with long-term impact, and individuals usually want to make these decisions for themselves. Competition, on the other hand, only intensifies in college.

Gender

There is a large literature which suggests that girls and boys, women and men, have had different experiences in science and mathematics in precollege and college. Is that true today, especially for men and women like those in this study? If there are differences, do they translate into different rates of persistence in premed or into different rates of acceptance to medical school? I will explore these questions for my sample of premed students.

Attraction to Medicine

The nature of the attraction to medicine is what the individual values personally about being a doctor. Those who are attracted to medicine for rewards that are not readily available from other occupations are likely to remain in premed longer than those whose attraction to medicine can be satisfied by other occupations. The strength or nature of the attraction to medicine can be the factor that differentiates the student with the B average in required premed courses who changes career goals from the similar student who continues in premed.

THE PROFESSION

Less than half of 1% of employed Americans are doctors (*Statistical Abstract*, 1991, p. 395). A minority of them are in private practice, and that number is likely to continue to decline. Yet job security and autonomy have long been major attractions for potential doctors. Twenty years ago premed students placed emphasis on "job security, prestige, being helpful to others, availability of job opportunities, working with people, and the opportunity to make an important contribution to society" (Hackman, Low-Beer, Wugmeister, Wilhelm, & Rosenbaum, 1979, p. 310). Now *managed care*, which is the latest organizational strategy of the health care industry, places controls on the professional activity and judgment of physicians, fewer of whom are engaged in a two-party relationship with their patients. Instead, physician and patient are two of the parties in a three-party relationship, where the third party is the health maintenance organization (HMO), or other insurer, or the government. Yet young women and men, hoping to be doctors in the near future, continue to exhibit idealism and commitment to human service goals and patient care that are threatened by these ongoing changes in the delivery of health care. They continue to value the autonomy projected in their image of a highly educated practicing professional. One student remarked: "I have a more realistic view [of medicine] now, but it is scary, with health reforms coming. Now it looks like we will all be working for someone else. I entered medicine in part to work independently."

For some students medicine is more than a career or even a profession; for them medicine is upward mobility. While Americans like to think of the United States as a classless society, this is not an accurate description. There is wide variation in household income, educational attainment, and occupation within the society. Entering an elite profession like medicine is one way for a young man or woman to have a more prosperous life and a more rewarding career than his or her parents had. For some of these individuals, the choice of premed as a college concentration initially was made for them by their parent(s) or at least was strongly reinforced by their parent(s). There is an added pressure on these premeds to succeed in gaining admission to medical school. For those who are upwardly mobile, it is not just the desire to help others, or the desire for a professional career, or even the desire for financial security that is the primary motivator. For them it is the combination of all of these elements and more in the profession of medicine that makes the goal so attractive and abandoning the goal so difficult.

In order for anyone to pursue this career path, she or he must follow a college preparatory science curriculum in high school. Quality as well as quantity in course offerings is important. While taking more science, especially biology, chemistry, and physics, is better than taking less, courses that teach scientific methodology and expose students to science's quantitative and research aspects are of greater value than courses that are largely descriptive, which teach *about* science rather than *doing* science. In college-level biology, "the emphasis now lies in determining critically and imaginatively what basic information is needed to define the key problems of living systems" (Hanson, 1969, p. 85). Nachtreib (1969) made a similar observation about chemistry, where "the questions have shifted from 'what' to 'why' and 'how' as the subject matter has deepened in theoretical and mathematical sophistication" (p. 98). Parents of today's high school and college students who took these courses when they were in college knew more about the periodic table weights and the physical properties of chemical substances, while students today know "much more about the forces that hold [substances] together and determine their molecular architecture" (p. 98).

OVERVIEW OF THIS BOOK

The remaining chapters of the book are devoted to preparation for medical school in a period of some institutional change for the profession. The focus of Chapter 2 is the profession of medicine as it has changed over time and its current standing as a rewarding profession with very competitive entrance requirements. Factors determining the selection of medical school applicants will be discussed, with particular reference to grades, standardized test scores, college or university attended, and the medical school interview. Some individual premed students are introduced in Chapter 2, and their progression through the premed process will be traced throughout the book. Chapter 3 introduces the process of occupational choice, with particular attention to the period before college. What are the various factors before college that influence the decisions of boys and girls to pursue medicine and the factors that affect their enrollment and performance in science courses? A modified rational choice perspective is applied to this decision process, and a descriptive model of the stages of occupational choice is used to interpret the ongoing choice process from childhood on. The relevant literature and the findings from this study pertaining to the precollege period will be discussed within the themes of academic factors, social factors, attraction to medicine, and gender.

Chapter 4 focuses on the college years, from the first to the last, on the decisions and experiences that move a person toward or away from the goal of medical school. The themes introduced in Chapter 3 will be pursued in Chapters 4 and 5. Chapter 5 concentrates on persistence and on the time of application and acceptance, on those choosing and those not choosing medical school, and on those chosen and not chosen. Chapter 6 looks forward and outward, with particular reference to the participants' views on the future of medicine and their role in it. With exposure to clinical practice through their volunteer work or paid employment in hospitals or with emergency medical services, they formed opinions of medical practice. In their college courses they became (more) familiar with the bigger picture of health care—changes in the practice of medicine, increased control by "third parties," and the economic factors that impact on the delivery of care. Chapter 6 includes some recommendations for those who want to achieve admission to medical school.

Chapter 2

THE PROFESSION OF MEDICINE

"Medical schools...are extremely risk-aversive in selecting members of their classes."
(Corder, 1994, p. 58)

The medical profession was upgraded significantly in the twentieth century, resulting in the requirement of higher qualifications and credentials to practice and in greater extrinsic rewards for physicians. The qualifications for *beginning* medical education have increased, too. While demonstrated achievement in the basic sciences is the primary selection criterion, even those students who earn above-average grades in science and mathematics courses are not guaranteed admission. Other aspects of their undergraduate education and life experience enhance or diminish their chances for admission to a medical school class.

THE DEVELOPMENT OF THE PROFESSION

The ongoing national debate on the cost and availability of health care is likely to result in far-reaching changes in the practice of medicine. Change is not new to medicine, however. The profession of medicine went through a major redefinition at the beginning of the twentieth century, when it inaugurated the professional training program and prerequisite science education that are taken for granted today. Throughout the nineteenth century, medical school was regarded as training that served as an alternative to the liberal arts; it was unusual that an individual would complete an undergraduate liberal arts curriculum and then go on to medical school. The admission requirement of an undergraduate degree added a credential to the process of medical training and enhanced the standing of the profession.

When the American Medical Association (AMA) was established in 1846, a primary purpose was "to raise and standardize the requirements for medical degrees" (Starr, 1982, p. 90). More than 60 years later, Flexner (1910) noted in his monumental study that medical students (in the sort of university-affiliated schools with which we are familiar today) needed sufficient background in biology, chemistry, and physics, instruction that went beyond that taught in most secondary schools. His report recommended that satisfactory completion of 2 years of college incorporating this curriculum should be made a minimum requirement for entry to medical school. At the time of the publication of his landmark report, only 16 medical schools then in existence in the United States and Canada met these criteria.

Flexner's work provided a comprehensive look at the state of medical education at that time. In 1893, Johns Hopkins University had established its medical school with an undergraduate degree as an entrance requirement. It was the first medical school to do so, and it was not until 1901 that Harvard Medical School imposed a similar qualification for admission. During the nineteenth century most medical schools in the United States were proprietary, offering lectures in combination with a period of apprenticeship with a practicing physician. Motivated by profit and not constrained by any national system of licensing or review, these schools, and the apprenticeships with which they were linked, varied greatly in their quality. Many had no laboratory facilities; that curriculum component was added later, when medical schools were more commonly affiliated with universities and with hospitals (Flexner, 1910). The link between medicine and science developed over time.

Acknowledgment of the *doctor* as a member of an elite profession did not originate with scientific medicine. Rather, it resulted from the recognition that doctors had knowledge of disease and its treatment that the general population lacked. Bullough (1966) noted that in the Middle Ages the body of medical knowledge was written in Latin, accessible only to those who could go through a period of long and difficult training.

Academic Preparation

For the past several decades the academic preparation required for a person to be accepted to medical school has not changed significantly. Today's standard premed curriculum had begun to emerge in the decade after the publication of the Flexner report. The following example was drawn from the 1920–21 catalog of one college for women: Premedical students should take general zoology, comparative anatomy of vertebrates, embryology, "and such other courses as time permits" (H. Sophie Newcomb, 1920, p. 59). In 1932–33, students interested in the natural sciences and premed students were required to take biology or chemistry or physics in the first year and two of these three subjects in the sophomore year; in the junior and senior years the student continued with one science for 4 years and a second science for 2 years (H. Sophie Newcomb, 1932). These science requirements were more stringent than the current premed curriculum. Today, only science majors would be likely to take courses in the same science discipline over 4 years. Premed requirements in the men's college in the same university were not so different, except that they took more science courses during the first 2 years (two each semester) and men interested in medicine were not required to earn the B.S. degree but could choose the B.A. instead (College of Arts and Sciences, 1932). In these early decades of the century, the supply of persons willing and able to undertake such a curriculum and, more important, of persons able to undertake a university degree program at all, was far more limited than today. In 1930, when the curriculum just described was in effect, 3.9% of the U.S. population had completed 4 or more years of college (Folger & Nam, 1967, p. 132); in 1989, in contrast, the number was 21% (*Statistical Abstract*, 1991, p. 38).

Costs

The scientific basis of medicine has resulted in limiting access to medical school to applicants who have demonstrated the appropriate aptitude and achievement in science. Costs, too, have kept out some potential doctors. Financial assistance for medical training, especially the government assistance available now through loans, is of relatively recent origin. Prior to these loan programs, it was very difficult for those lacking substantial family resources to become doctors. Even today, cost is a major issue for many would-be doctors. One student in our study who was accepted to more than one medical school but selected his state school instead of a private, out-of-state university said that he was told that it would cost $50,000 a year to go to the private institution.

Medical School Accreditation

After requirements for medical school admission were standardized, the AMA took on new challenges, resulting in the association's increased control over the profession. This control was manifested in the authority to accredit medical schools, the so-called *gatekeeping* function, which it shares with the Association of American Medical Colleges (AAMC) in a joint body, the Liaison Committee on Medical Education (LCME). The gatekeeper grants or limits access, in this case by controlling the number of medical schools that may operate in the United States. While each institution sets the size of its medical school, based on its faculty size and composition and by its laboratory and other facilities, final approval to operate a medical school of a particular size must be given by the LCME. Accreditation is renewed (or not) every 7 years (Liaison Committee in Medical Education, 1995). Because the class size is set, each school monitors its admissions process carefully. In order for students and the medical school to receive federal funds, including student loans, the school must be accredited. Furthermore, only graduates of accredited medical schools may take the U.S. Medical Licensing Exam (USMLE). Students from foreign medical schools who want to obtain a medical residency in the United States must complete a certification process consisting of a passing score on a proficiency test in English, a passing score on the USMLE, and an evaluation of their educational records and curriculum. In this era of intense competition for entry, one of the accrediting criteria is more easily met than others: "To achieve and maintain accreditation, each medical school must demonstrate that it has access to a pool of applicants sufficiently large and possessing national level qualifications to fill its first year class" (AAMC, 1995, p. 16). No medical school today suffers from a shortage of applicants.

Licensing

The distinction between who is a doctor and who is not provides the profession with autonomy, as nonpractitioners lack the knowledge required to evaluate or criticize the doctor (Freidson, 1970). Unlike other healers, doctors are licensed by the state, and unlicensed individuals who engage in the practice of medicine can be fined or sent to jail. M. Friedman (1962) made a distinction between occupations that restrict entry to practice but not to training programs and those, like medicine, that severely restrict entry to the training programs necessary to practice. Entry into the occupation is likely to happen eventually in the former but not in the latter.

The licensure and regulation of the medical profession sends the message to the general public that only those individuals who have successfully completed the appropriate scientific training will be permitted to apply what they have learned to the treatment of disease. One reason that licensing became necessary was that doctors in one state might have received their training in a medical school in another part of the country, in a school with which individuals in this state might have been unfamiliar (Ludmerer, 1983). Licensing insured that certain standards were met nationwide. While it may be difficult to understand now that persons in Florida might be suspicious of doctors trained to practice medicine in Illinois or New York, that is because licensing has been in effect for many years. Earlier in this century, when medical training was also offered by proprietary schools and other programs not directly connected to universities, high-quality outcomes could not be taken for granted. With licensing, however, the patients of doctors were expected to have faith in science and trust that a licensed physician was using his or her training correctly. This view of medicine as applied science has prevailed throughout much of the present century. States still wield some influence in the licensing process, however; while all states use the USMLE, each state sets its own standard for a passing grade.

Doctor–Patient Relationship

Restrictions on the number of physicians and the corresponding power of the professional association to enforce these restrictions result in benefits to individual physicians, including high salaries and job security, and some control over the doctor–patient relationship. As long ago as 1847 the Code of Ethics of the AMA referred to the mutual obligations of physician and patient: "One prominent theme . . . was that patients should be totally loyal to the physician or find another doctor" (Berlant, 1975, p. 114). While Berlant noted that this stipulation was omitted from the revised code of 1903, there is evidence that this issue is again prompting concern among physicians. Some individuals today join HMOs because their employers provide incentives to do so or because they realize personal cost savings. At the same time, they may wish to maintain a consultative or even a treatment relationship with the independent physician who used to treat them. Such a nonexclusive arrangement is not always acceptable to the primary care physician in the HMO, who may insist on an exclusive relationship with his or her patients (Rosenthal, 1994).

There is some tension between the doctor's scientific training and the role of caregiver. Critics in the medical profession and among the premed population say that too little attention is given to the personal and human aspects and demands of the doctor–patient relationship. A majority of individuals pursuing the study of medicine are doing so to serve humankind, while recognizing also that the medical profession is an especially demanding one as practiced within the context of medicine-as-business. While the growth of HMOs has increased the patient load for many doctors, Shryock noted that the task of accommodating a large number of patients is not of recent origin:

> "The average of my private patients in the late summer and fall months," wrote a physician in 1849, "is generally between 30 and 40 (per day) and to get through with these . . . I am going round from sunrise to 9 or 10 o'clock at night." In addition, he saw daily 60 to 70 hospital patients. (Shryock, 1928, quoted in Shryock, 1966, p. 164)

SOME REWARDS OF MEDICINE

The rewards that medicine offers to practitioners are intrinsic and extrinsic. The intrinsic rewards include those directly involved in the practice of medicine—doing good for others, challenge, autonomy, among others. Extrinsic rewards such as income and prestige follow from the practice of medicine. Sociological research on occupational rewards has concentrated more on extrinsic rewards, which are more easily measured.

Prestige

The attractiveness of an occupation may be evaluated by its social standing, the respect that members of this occupation are given by individuals throughout the society. National rankings of occupational prestige are constructed periodically from surveys of cross-sections of the U.S. population. While such rankings are by no means exact, it is possible to identify some dimensions used by individuals to measure standing. One factor is autonomy, the degree to which those in the occupation work without supervision. Other factors include the amount and difficulty of the education or other training required to learn the occupation, the perceived importance of the tasks, especially the consequences of the practitioner's actions for the life, health, safety, and liberty of others. Another item for this list of factors affecting the assignment of prestige to individual occupations is the lack of visible corruption in the occupation or industry overall.

As noted in Chapter 1, when national samples of American adults are questioned about the social standing of occupations, with extraordinary consistency they put *physician* at the top of the scale. One study compared three rankings that measured prestige in different ways. *Physician* topped all three (Bose, 1985). Consequently, those individuals interested in recognition from others will find few substitutes for the profession of medicine.

An anomalous contributing factor to an occupation's prestige is the degree to which performance of tasks involves getting soiled: Is getting one's hands or clothing dirty or stained a regular part of the job? Flexner (1910) noted that before surgery was based on biological science and an understanding of the systems of the body, surgeons learned from experience—their own and that of others. They often applied general remedies, such as bleeding, in an attempt to treat a patient. Consequently, surgeons were regarded as having less prestige than other doctors. With the advent of science-based medicine and the extensive training required to specialize in surgery, surgeons now receive higher salaries and prestige than most other medical specialists and nonspecialists.

Income

Salary data for the various medical specialties demonstrate that the *average* salaries in medicine, across specialties, are likely to be very competitive with those of any profession. Although an entrepreneur, high-level business executive, or Wall Street attorney may earn more than a physician, even one with a specialized practice, it is the expected earnings, the average earnings of that profession, that will be the more relevant consideration in the choice of occupation. And there are few average earnings higher than those in medicine. One source reported a *low* average of $119,000 for family practitioners, $310,000 for radiologists, and $575,000 for cardiac surgeons in private practice (Eckholm, 1993, p. 1). Another source reports somewhat lower figures: $92,000–$103,000 for primary care physicians and $163,000–$188,000 for specialists (Corder, 1994, p. 3).

More surprising may be the age at which these occupational rewards are first recognized. Goldstein and Oldham (1979) reported on the income estimates provided by grade school children for selected occupations; doctors' salaries were always among the highest. First-grade girls estimated that doctors earned $41 per year, compared with boys' estimate of $50, and both figures were *higher* than incomes estimated for other occupations. By grade 7, girls' estimates of physicians' income had reached $30,000 and boys', $23,000 (rounded); by this time, "only the President of the U.S. ranked higher than doctor" (p. 58).

The conventional wisdom within the profession, to which premed students are exposed, is that salaries will decline substantially in the coming years. This is a prediction, however, rather than a fact. At best this prediction introduces uncertainty into an individual's calculation of trade-offs—at what point will he or she be able to pay off medical school debts and enjoy higher financial rewards? At worst, for the individual whose motivation is primarily economic, the concern that medicine could fail to deliver a highly valued reward would make it a less attractive occupation.

Why are doctors paid so well? One explanation for these high salaries is contained in the functionalist argument, articulated in 1945 by sociologists K. Davis and Moore. Briefly stated, those occupations that contribute the most to the functioning of the society *and* that also require the greatest training are those that are rewarded most highly. So, while it is very important to the overall society that trash be collected at frequent intervals, the amount of training required to become a trash collector is comparatively low. A physician, on the other hand, is a person to whom we entrust our lives. It is a profession that requires extensive training in order to perform a difficult and stressful job. The monetary rewards, therefore, are paid in recognition of the physician's value to society and in compensation for the length and cost of the training involved. If there were no high salaries for doctors, the argument posits, premeds would not work as hard as they do in college to achieve at the level necessary for admission to medical school. Nor would they continue to labor and give up other activities—sleep, income, and leisure—or bear the costs of very high tuition. The financial rewards act as incentives to endure the training period. This summary of the functionalist position directs attention to the financial and prestige rewards of occupations, which are more easily measured and compared than more intangible intrinsic rewards.

While the premeds in my study may have been unaware of this sociological theory, some of them nevertheless expressed in functional terms their concern that any move toward socialized medicine would reduce the financial rewards to individual doctors.

> People want the best health care available but don't want to pay. Doctors should make a lot; the job is difficult and the training is demanding.

> The cost of medical education is extremely high. Residents don't make much and then you have lots of loans to pay back. With cost containment in the future, doctors will not make as much.

> As a freshman, I didn't know what was going on. Now I know there will be changes, [including] less income; if my income [as a doctor] were $60,000, is it worth it? There should be more medical schools.

> I disagree with HMOs and any kind of socialized medicine. You are dealing with people [doctors] who control your life. If they want to charge $100,000,000 to pull a tooth, they should be allowed to do so. There is more stress for premeds, medical students, and doctors than for other professions, and doctors should be compensated. Students who take out loans for college and medical school are counting on that income to pay the loans.

Conflict theory, an alternative explanation for the high monetary rewards for doctors, focuses on the competition among occupational groups for scarce resources. There is a finite amount of money available to be expended in salaries, and those occupational groups with more power can command a larger portion of these scarce resources than groups with less power. (A thorough treatment of the conflict perspective can be found in Dahrendorf, 1959.) Conflict theory can be used to explain why two occupations at the same level of skill and training receive very discrepant levels of average salary/wages: One occupation is highly organized, in a union, and the other is not. When the union can threaten to withhold the services of its members if wages or salaries are not increased, it is likely that compensation in this occupation will increase more than in a similar occupation that is not organized. The union serves to reduce the discrepancy in power between workers and management.

While doctors are not unionized, they do benefit from the strength of a professional association, the American Medical Association. With power to limit the number of doctors who will be educated, the AMA, with the AAMC, has the power to influence salaries in the profession. Although my study participants were not asked a question that would directly test their understanding of this power of the AMA, a few respondents volunteered their views. For example: "In high school I didn't have a good picture of the physician as part of a big organization, the AMA.[Now I know that] physicians lobby for things through the AMA."

Autonomy and Security

There are other rewards that distinguish medicine from most other occupations. Autonomy and security, in particular, are identified as attractions to the profession of medicine. The U.S. labor force has been undergoing a transformation: The number of management positions is declining in many industries, as organizations *streamline* and *downsize*. Insecurity derives from the ever-present probability that skills that have been regarded as valuable and practiced only by those with extensive training are being incorporated into more sophisticated computer software. To further exacerbate matters, men and women completing higher education today enter a labor force that is dominated by members of the baby-boom cohort. As if a shrinking supply of opportunities across many fields were not enough, people born between the late 1940s and the early 1960s are in the middle-management and higher-management positions that the younger cohort will want to enter before the older group will be willing to vacate them.

Where does this leave those who want to be doctors? They see many of their college peers worrying about long-term career prospects in other fields. To a lesser extent, they, too, are concerned. Beyond the premed anxiety about getting into medical school is the concern that the proposed measures to cut costs in the health care industry will result in changes in the practice of medicine. Fewer doctors will be attending to more patients, in managed-care situations. Yet once licensed to practice, doctors still enjoy more security than most other professionals. Potential doctors compete for entrée to the education for their profession, while in other professions the competition is later, for positions. These other professionals live increasingly with the fear that they could be out of work. While few doctors expect to lose their positions, they perceive a different threat to the practice of their profession as they would choose to practice it—the loss of autonomy. The move toward greater management of care is the move toward more health care provided in HMOs and less in private practices. Several premed students spoke in the interviews about wanting a family practice in a small-town or rural setting. For many, this was a statement of their preference for autonomy.

MEDICAL SCHOOL ADMISSION CRITERIA

The premed experience, in total, is preliminary socialization to an elite profession that brings high levels of reward. A part of the premed experience is told with numbers, as is most often the case when there are more applicants than positions or more buyers than sellers. In order to differentiate among applicants, the admissions committees in medical schools will use some quantifiable criteria. Specifically, they use undergraduate (and sometimes graduate) overall cumulative grade-point average, grades in the required premed science courses (and possibly all science courses completed), and scores on the subtests of the Medical College Admission Test subtests (MCAT). Applicants who score high on all three measures make the first cut; those high on two and low(er) on one may get another look. Medical schools can also restrict access to the application process: One student reported that "some medical schools do not give you an application if your MCAT scores are low."

The policies of undergraduate institutions also influence the degree to which the medical school application process is open to all premed students. At some colleges and universities, students will not receive an institutional recommendation or a practice interview if their GPA and their MCAT scores do not suggest they have a reasonable chance of admission. Other institutions, including the one where I conducted my study, open the process to all who have completed premed requirements and the MCAT. High school students visiting colleges can ask about the institution's practice. After learning what proportion of last year's premed seniors was admitted to medical school, they can ask whether the population of students referred to includes all who had completed premed requirements (including MCAT) and were interested in medical school or only those whose GPA and MCAT performances had reached some minimally acceptable level set by the undergraduate institution. The admission rate obviously will be higher in the second type of school, because the students with weaker profiles have been eliminated. Yet the occasional student whose record is borderline does get admitted, because the admissions committee finds merit in her or his total application and interview. This slim chance for admission evaporates for the marginal applicant who does not have an institutional recommendation from his or her university. While a student may apply without such a recommendation, this is uncommon and may raise a red flag to the admissions committee.

Some men and women do persist in a premed program when their grades are comparatively low. Others with higher grades still question their ability. Some love science and are torn between scientific research and medicine. Others take as few science courses as possible, major in a nonscience subject, and are impatient for the clinical training they will receive in their later years in medical school. Some change their focus while in college, as this student did: "I am less oriented toward research now and more clinically oriented. I am also concerned that this limits the amount of change I can effect." No premed student need be unaware of the requirements for entrance to medical school, the *what* that needs to be done. More elusive is a good understanding of the process, the *how*. There is no formula for reaching the goal. There are some general contributing factors, and there are differing manifestations of each factor. And, unfortunately for those who seek a single truth, there are exceptions. While no one save a genius wants to learn that some students find the courses and the MCAT to be *easy* and the medical school interviews enjoyable, such students do exist. For example: "I never thought of premed as scary or demanding. I never felt a strong bond with 'the suffering premeds.'" For most students, however, the program is difficult: "I have a lot more respect [now] for what doctors went through to get where they are."

Coursework and Grades

The prerequisite courses for medical school are taken over a 3-year period, and most premed students take additional science courses beyond the prerequisites. All premeds must take two semesters of general chemistry, two semesters of biology, two semesters of organic chemistry, two semesters of physics, and one or two semesters of mathematics, which often includes calculus. The mathematics requirement is specified by the individual medical schools. The eight science courses have laboratory components associated with them, of 3–4 hours per lab per week, for a total of 6–7 classroom hours per week per course. The AAMC specifies that the science and mathematics courses "should be rigorous and, in general, acceptable for students majoring in those areas" (*Medical School Admission Requirements*, 1991, p. 15).

While some students take one or more of their science courses during the summer, this is not always a good decision. Medical schools want evidence that a prospective medical student can perform well in a science-intensive curriculum. They want to see that applicants took two science prerequisite courses with labs in at least 1 year, rather than taking one during the summer. If students must take one of the courses during the summer, while doubling up in another year, they are advised to take the course at their university or at a college or university at least as demanding as their home institution. Medical school admissions staff are quite skilled at reading transcripts and at reading between the lines as well.

The required sequence of premed courses is regarded as difficult largely because understanding in these fields is cumulative. If a student fails to grasp the fundamental concepts, he or she cannot succeed in courses later in the sequence. The first courses in these science sequences are described as *beginning* or *general* in college catalogs, yet the labeling can mislead students who are prepared for a lengthy review of high school science. The pace of college courses is swift, with more analysis, more calculation, and less description. There is a lot more information presented in each course and higher expectations from instructors of how much will be retained. "The teacher taught to the top of the class," one premed reported. Another noted that "courses in college [do] start from scratch and novices can do well, but the tests in chemistry and biology are much more difficult in college." Specific comparisons between high school and college courses were described as follows:

> There are 30 problems per chapter and two chapters per week; it is hard to get to them all.

> The pace in chemistry is unreal. All that I learned in high school chemistry was covered in 2 weeks here.

> Everything I learned in 2 years of high school chemistry was covered on my first test [in college chemistry].

> Things I covered in my high school [chemistry] course were covered in one sentence here.

One student described the differences between her small high school and her college experience this way:

> In high school, the teachers walked you through, held your hand, made sure you understood. Here, professors don't care—you must do it all yourself. That's the way it should be, actually, because throughout your life you will not have someone being sure you are doing what you should.

But some of their fellow students came to college with particularly strong high school preparation:

The first semester of college chemistry was similar to high school chemistry.

A lot of General Chemistry I was review for me.

My high school [chemistry] course was similar to college; we had to work problems in high school, too.

Students who completed 2 years of chemistry while in high school and then enrolled in the first chemistry course in college would be expected to have an advantage over their fellow students, most of whom took only one year of chemistry in high school. This advantage did not always translate into a high grade in general chemistry, however. Some of these students acknowledged that they destroyed their advantage by becoming so overconfident that they devoted too little time to the course. Another explanation was suggested by students' perceptions of differences between high school and college-level science courses—in the content, volume, and presentation of material. A similar situation is encountered in medical school. With a faster pace of courses or a perspective quite different from that of the college courses, students who studied the subject in college will have little or no advantage over other students.

In the premed program the pace picks up even more in the advanced courses beyond General Chemistry. Those students who can keep up are those who are most likely to succeed in the long run. While this observation may seem trivial, it is not. Success in the premed curriculum involves more than attending class, taking notes, and reading the assigned texts. It means concentrating while in class, absorbing enough from classes and reading to apply material to new situations, and remembering enough to use this acquired knowledge in next semester's and next year's courses. Becker, Geer, Hughes, and Strauss (1961) noted that "uncritical learning, memorizing really, presents itself as a way of covering the work when there isn't time to think about it" (p. 97). Yet the content of science courses becomes increasingly abstract, so an understanding of the basic concepts is far more useful than an attempt to memorize discrete bits of information. In medical school, the pace is even quicker and the formal evaluations (examinations) even less frequent. While at least one school is moving toward more frequent testing (Robbins et al., 1995), this is not the norm. The quantity of information presented in the basic sciences can be overwhelming, especially for students who try to understand and absorb all of the new information as it is being presented. There is no value in adopting the attitude that one will study the material tomorrow, as there will be just as much additional new information to learn then.

Medical school curricula differ to some degree across institutions, but generally they consist of 2 years of a medical science curriculum—the required courses and some specialized elective options—followed by 2 years of clinical work. The clinical aspects of medicine are introduced during the first 2 years, so that students see the relationship between the two components of the curriculum. Completing some specialized science courses while in college does not necessarily result in higher grades when taking courses in these subjects during the first 2 years of medical school (Canaday & Lancaster, 1985). The explanation for this lack of association is not straightforward. It may be, as these authors suggested, that students who have a background in biochemistry or anatomy, for example, feel that they have an advantage over other students in the class and therefore do not put as much study time into the course. They choose instead to devote this time to other subjects. This interpretation is consistent with findings from our interviews.

Becker and colleagues (1961) noted of students entering medical school in 1956: "All but a few had attained an average of B or higher in their college work" (p. 10). A comparison of applications made during the 1960s with those of the 1970s shows that while 31% of applicants to medical school in the 1970s had college grade-point averages between 3.60 and 4.00, only 17% had these grades during the 1960s (D. G. Johnson, 1983, p. 55). While some readers might see this as an indicator of grade inflation during the later period, it is also the result of increased competition. Johnson went on to say that "by the end of the decade of the 1970s, approximately half of all medical school entrants had grade averages in the 'A' range" (p. 55). A study of medical school applicants during the early 1980s reported that roughly a third had cumulative grade-point averages and science grade-point averages in excess of 3.50 (Tudor & Beran, 1987, p. 562). The mean undergraduate GPA of entrants for the 1993 entering class was 3.47, and 3.26 for all applicants (AAMC, 1994b).

> In recent years those individuals admitted with less than a 3.00 GPA have either achieved strikingly improved performances in their later years of college or demonstrated other characteristics deemed desirable by the various medical school admission committees. (*Medical School Admission Requirements*, 1991, p. 17)

Institutional Quality

An admissions factor that seldom is made explicit but that has influence in admissions decisions is the selectivity of the applicant's undergraduate institution. In our interviews this issue was raised often by students who had made informal comparisons of their premed courses and course examinations with those of their friends at other universities where entrance requirements were lower. One student in the study, who had transferred from another university during her freshman year, reported that the premed courses at her new university were much more difficult than those she had taken at her previous institution. She was able to make a direct comparison because she had completed the first semester of a year-long course prior to transferring. Once registered for the second semester, she felt underprepared to continue the course, having covered far less material in the first semester than was covered by students who had completed the first semester at her current institution.

There is some evidence to support the belief that students graduating from more highly selective institutions (which accept a smaller percentage of applicants and have higher entrance requirements) are more likely to be admitted to medical school, other things equal or nearly so, than those from less selective colleges. According to Bartlett (1969), "with the notable exception of a few small, selective liberal arts colleges, it is the large, well-established universities which are preparing students for medical school" (p. 130). Lewis (1984), too, noted a disproportionate representation of applicants from the more prestigious categories of undergraduate institutions, using Carnegie Commission categories. There is evidence of a *charter* effect here (Meyer, 1972), a widespread understanding that certain institutions or types of institution produce in their graduates recognizable and valued outcomes. Students in college and those anticipating attending college, too, are aware of these effects. At college information sessions held with high school students and their parents a frequently asked question of the college's representative is the acceptance rates of their graduates to medical and law schools. One of the premeds put it this way:

> You never feel you will be accepted into medical school. The fact that I attended this university was a help in dental school admission. They recognized that I attended a very competitive school, where Bs and Cs may have been As at other schools.

Jones and Adams (1983) noted that some medical schools weigh college cumulative grade-point averages by the selectivity of the institution. Such weighting of academic record by school quality must be done by the individual medical schools if it is to be done at all. Clapp and Reid (1976) noted that the American College Application Service (AMCAS) does not weigh GPA by institution.

F. R. Hall and Bailey (1992) looked at the relationship between the quality of the medical student's undergraduate college and the student's academic performance in the first year of medical school. They noted that students entering from colleges or universities with low average SATs had higher undergraduate science GPAs than those coming from more selective institutions. Students from more competitive institutions may be accepted with lower grades. The authors found no significant differences between the two groups in grades at the end of the first year in medical school, however, suggesting that a medical school can admit students with lower grades from higher-ranking schools and still see success. Jones and Adams (1983) examined the relationship between science GPA in college and scores on MCAT science subtests. Students with the highest science grades from less selective colleges and universities tended to score lower on the MCAT. Students with lower science GPAs (B to B+) from the most competitive schools were equal on their MCAT scores only with A students from less selective institutions. F. R. Hall and Bailey (1992) found that "MCAT scores and [college] GPAs become more valid predictors when college selectivity is used as a weighing factor" (p. 5).

Meyer's (1972) analysis of how institutional characteristics affect outcomes for students by validating their experience differs from earlier scholarship on the effects of college attended on individual student achievement. What is the value to a person of having attended a college that ranks highly? One perspective on this issue is described as the *frog pond* effect (J. A. Davis, 1967). In a pond of big frogs, only a bigger frog is the really *big* frog. The level of competition within highly selective colleges has a negative effect on outcomes; students who were strong in high school will earn lower grades in college. To earn a degree from such an institution, many graduates will have sacrificed the higher grades they could have earned at a less selective school. One premed student expressed concern, describing "a drowning feeling that you can't compete with all of the people in your classes. In a good school where everyone is intelligent, you must compete with each other and all courses [in premed] are graded on a curve." The effect levels out only if the graduate or professional school or the employer takes into account the college's reputation rather than assuming that grades are equivalent across schools.

The frog pond is contrasted with another model, that of *environmental press*, which posits the opposite effect: A college's selectivity in admission "should positively affect aspirations [of enrolled students], since an undergraduate will perform best and aim highest at a school where most of his fellow students have high aspirations and are superior academically" (Drew & Astin, 1972, p. 1152).

Interview results from this study and those from work cited here suggest an answer to the question: Is it better to be one of the top students in a less selective college or a less outstanding student in a more selective college? It is *best* for the individual wishing to go on to medical school to be a high performer in a highly ranked college. The risk involved in attending the less selective college is that of being affected negatively by the lower level of competition. No one can count on being at the top, especially if they need the stimulation of difficult courses and very talented competition in order to reach their potential. Yet the students who perform less well in comparison with other students in the class will still receive low grades, even at the most highly selective of colleges. These individuals may take some consolation in knowing that their competition was more difficult than for students at lesser-ranked schools and that medical schools may take institutional quality into account. They know, too, that medical schools will limit the allowance that they give to this factor. Given the combined risks of not rising to the top of the class and, if they do, of having their accomplishment evaluated within the context of a less selective college and curriculum, future premeds should matriculate at a more selective institution if possible.

MCAT Scores

Unlike more general aptitude tests, such as the SAT, which tests knowledge of and facility with English vocabulary and grammar and basic mathematical concepts, the MCAT tests scientific knowledge and the ability to apply this knowledge in solving problems, as well as command of English and writing ability, all in one day-long set of tests. The current version of the test includes four subtests: the verbal and the two science subtests (in multiple-choice format), and the essay component. The multiple-choice sections are scored from 1 to 15; scores in the double digits are considered high. In 1992–93, 30% of men and 19% of women scored 10 or higher on the biological sciences subtest. Corresponding percentages for the physical sciences subtest were 23% and 14.5% and for the verbal reasoning subtest, 26% and 26% (AAMC, 1994a, p. 27). The gender gap was smaller on all subtests than was observed among test-takers a decade earlier, with a previous version of the test. While the percentage scoring 10 or higher on subtests has declined for both men and women as the number of applicants has increased, applicants are not required to score in the double digits. A representative of one private university's medical school admissions committee told me, "It is difficult for us to accept a student whose MCAT in the sciences is less than 8. On the other hand, we find little difference between scores of 9 and 13."

Some premeds who scored highly on the MCAT subtests reported that the test covered only the basic information taught in the required premed science courses. Those who scored lower were more inclined to emphasize the difficulty of the test and the more-than-basic knowledge the test was measuring. They often said they wished they had taken more science courses. While it may be the case that a particular course in physiology or genetics would have helped in answering a few more questions correctly, there is no evidence that simply taking more science courses will improve performance. There are students who, having mastered the basics, did well on the test even though they majored in a subject other than those covered in the science subtests and took few biological or physical science courses beyond those required. Successful completion of courses in humanities and social sciences can result in an improvement in the verbal or writing components of the MCAT as well as demonstrating a wide range of interests that medical schools find attractive (Olmstead & Sheffrin, 1981). More specifically, verbal scores are associated with analytical ability (Elam & Johnson, 1997b).

Students whose scores are low often decide to retake the test, which is offered twice a year. Some medical schools will not ignore the earlier scores, but they will also take the new scores into account. Other schools use only the most recent scores, although that practice is not common (Mitchell, 1987). Students whose scores are *borderline* have a more difficult decision to make: If they retake the MCAT and earn a lower score on the retake, they have hurt their chances for admission to those schools that count only the most recent scores or that average together both sets of scores. Although some applicants would like to diminish the emphasis placed on the MCAT, at least one study has found that the correlation between MCAT scores and performance in the first year of medical school was even higher than that between science GPA and medical school performance (M. L. Hall & Stocks, 1995).

The MCAT is a key factor in the screening of applicants, but it is not the only important factor. Students who have accumulated good grades in a wider variety of subjects than sciences alone have broader knowledge and skills to apply to test and interview situations. Students who choose a nonscience discipline as their major field while also pursuing a premed curriculum are not relying on a science major to get them into medical school. While a science major can help on the MCAT, some premeds who choose biology as a major are weaker students who select this major because they hope it will prove advantageous when they take the MCAT and apply to medical school. That medical schools may respond to a choice of major was experienced directly by one student: "Many who interviewed me welcomed my liberal arts background. My English major helped me to think critically." In 1992 and 1993, 57% of MCAT examinees were biological science majors (AAMC, 1994a). Another source notes that while biology is the major chosen most often by students intending to pursue careers in medicine and other health sciences, "the acceptance rate of biology majors [to medical school] is slightly less than average" (Corder, 1994, p. 6).

Johnson, in his study of medical students from 1950 to 1980, found that those who were admitted to medical school with *average* MCAT scores and a C+ cumulative grade-point average in college completed medical school in the usual 4 years (cited in McGaghie, 1990). This study could not be replicated today, as the criteria in use would not produce a sufficient sample of C+ students who had been admitted. Johnson's conclusion—that medical schools could increase the weight of criteria other than grades and test scores in making their selection among applicants—would come as a great relief to some of today's applicants who are involved actively in community service with the Red Cross or in hospital emergency rooms, or who are employed as emergency medicine technicians and phlebotomists. However, it would make the selection process more subjective and consequently more difficult to predict who would get in and who would be left out. While some students who had accumulated the record of experience just described would get in, provided their science grades and MCAT scores were *good enough*, there still would be far more applicants than spaces for them. This change in selection procedure would only substitute a new set of disappointed applicants for those we have now, and some *qualified* applicants still would be denied. Only one out of two or three individuals applying to medical school is accepted using the current criteria for science achievement. Without such quantifiable measures of past successes, selection would become more random as it became more subjective. There has been some call for change:

> Too often, small differences in scores on the examinations [MCAT] are used to differentiate among candidates with comparable academic qualifications and, thus, to make final selection decisions. This represents an inappropriate emphasis on an instrument that is designed to assess only part of the students' overall qualifications to study medicine. (Muller, 1984, p. 9)

There is no evidence, however, that such reservations have been heard; indeed, the MCAT has been redesigned to measure a wider range of achievements and, with more applicants per opening, it is likely that more, not less, emphasis will be placed on these tests. Medical schools want well-rounded students, not individuals whose only interest is science. Yet they continue to place the greater weight of their decision on science performance and look at other interests and achievements only among those applicants who have already excelled in the requisite science courses and the MCAT.

The Interview

After demonstrating superior academic credentials and before an applicant is admitted, she or he must be interviewed. Some of the rejected applicants present poor credentials overall: a low grade-point average in college, low grades in required science and math courses, and low scores on the MCAT subtests. These individuals will not progress to the second stage of the application process, where an admissions committee looks beyond these numbers—to involvement and leadership in college organizations, to commitment to medicine through community service and scientific research experience, and to the application essay. Applicants whose academic records as measured by grades and test scores demonstrate a higher level of achievement will get a second look. At that time, letters of recommendation and experience in out-of-class activities related to medicine's clinical or research aspects become important and may result in an interview.

The interview usually involves a trip to the campus of the medical school and a meeting with the admissions committee. While some schools will conduct interviews in other locations, this is not a common occurrence, creating a hardship for students who do not have and cannot borrow the necessary travel funds to visit one or more schools. "I had [offers of] interviews at two schools . . . but I couldn't go because of money. A regional interview was an option at one of the schools but not at the other." (This student was subsequently admitted to a third school.)

During the interview, members of the committee ask the questions and the candidate responds. It is common for the candidate to meet separately with one or more members of the admissions committee who have access to the candidate's file and with one or two other individuals—members of the faculty or a faculty member and a student—who do not have access to the file. A tour of the facilities and an opportunity to meet some current students may be included. The content of the interview is more difficult to specify, as the format and questions asked of applicants vary across schools. Some of the premeds reported that their annual interviews for this project were good preparation for the medical school interview, as there was some (unintentional) overlap in the sets of questions. When representatives of medical school admissions staffs were asked what they look for in candidates during the interview process, a majority of them reported "motivation and interest in medical school," "interpersonal skills and character," "maturity," and "evidence of extra-curricular activities" (E. K. Johnson & Edwards, 1991, p. 410). Interviewers are more likely to ask about opinions, values, and goals than to ask questions that have less ambiguous right and wrong answers. While the percentage of completed applications that result in interviews varies across schools, it hardly ever reaches one in three and may be as low as one in six. An approximate ratio of applicants interviewed to those accepted to the first-year class is three-to-one.

Shaw, Martz, Lancaster, and Sade (1995), reporting on a survey by Johnson and Edwards of all U. S. medical schools, said that "the primary purpose of the interview . . . was to assess noncognitive skills" (p. 532). Yet their own study of interviews conducted at one medical school found that the applicant's college grade-point average was the largest influence on the interviewer's rating of noncognitive traits. These results suggest that the interview as an admission factor is not as independent of the applicant's academic performance as some hope it will be.

One participant in this study was pretty certain that her written response to a question posed on the application form, asking her to enumerate weaknesses that might impact on her performance in medical school and in the practice of medicine, was responsible for her failure to get an interview at that school. While her grades were excellent, in science and in nonscience courses alike, and her scores on the MCAT were at least above average, her essay, written with great humility, focused on her concern that she might not be good enough to be a doctor. Her own idealism about medicine and her feelings of awe combined with personal insecurity may have cost her the interview. In one study of premed students, "48% of females (compared to 58% of males) say that they are 'very sure' they have what it takes to be a good doctor" (Fiorentine, 1988, p. 244). The remaining 52% of women and 42% of men either questioned their ability or lacked confidence in it. While insecurity is not an uncommon product of premedical education, admitting its existence during the application process can bring negative results.

From the Medical School's Perspective

Admissions committee chairs or representatives at eight medical schools, public and private, were interviewed for this study. These individuals were asked: Which factors are weighed most heavily when you are considering applicants for admission to (your) medical school? Not all of these schools had a formal system of weighing criteria, and those that had such a system did not always agree on what was most important. There was agreement among respondents that MCAT and science GPA carried the most weight, followed by cumulative GPA, extracurricular activities, difficulty of course load, and community service. Their responses include:

> We give equal consideration to the academic and nonacademic side. On the academic side we look for adequate preparation to handle medical school. One must do reasonably well in premed courses and on the MCAT, with grades weighed more heavily. With 5,000 to 6,000 applications, 3,000 to 4,000 are reasonable, using these criteria.

For that school, college attended was not an important factor, because "some students do not have the option of going to a better school."

Thinking that one school [college] is better than others leads us into problems. A student should do well at whatever school he or she chooses. Letters of recommendation are important, as is the interview. We expect you to have a good interview; if you do not, that is bad.

All things being equal, the higher the MCAT score, the greater the probability of acceptance. A strong MCAT score can offset a modest GPA, but not the reverse. MCAT measures retention of and the ability to use information. If there is any disparity of grades across subjects contributing to the GPA, the science grades are more important. Students should get some hospital experience. We want concern for others to come out in a student. We try to select those applicants who will make the best physicians, not those who will make the best medical students.

We screen applicants on MCAT, cumulative GPA, GPA in the required premed courses, and college attended. Students from less competitive colleges may have higher grades; then we would downgrade the importance of GPA and place more emphasis on the MCAT. Students have to absorb a lot [in their premed courses] that they may not understand and hence they must memorize some things. Organic chemistry is the course most like medical school coursework.

If we are familiar with the undergraduate college, then the GPA from that school will carry weight. If we know that grades from a particular school tend to be inflated, or if we have less experience with that school, then MCAT will carry more weight.... One needs a certain level of academic performance to get a foot in the door. Then, well-roundedness becomes important.

One student who had been interviewed added:

We are told in medical school interviews that the emphasis is not so much on grades or scores, because everyone [everyone selected for an interview] has those. Now dedication and the desire to serve come into play.

Mitchell (1987), reporting on a 1986 survey of personnel in 113 medical schools, had similar findings: The most important factors in admission were "overall science undergraduate GPA, quality of the degree-granting institution, letters of evaluation, interview ratings, MCAT scores, extracurricular activities, work in areas related to health care, breadth and/or difficulty of course work, and state of legal residence" (p. 871). She reported that a number of medical schools in her survey had changed (presumably increasing) their weighing of MCAT data for applicants from unfamiliar institutions.

Data from as early as the 1970s showed that private universities with medical schools supplied a disproportionate number of recent college graduates who were admitted to medical schools (Tidball, 1985). More recently, according to Corder (1994), "there are no data to show this [completing undergraduate work at an institution with a medical school] to make any significant difference in your chances for admission" (p. 5). There is not likely to be an aggregate difference, but the connection within a university can indeed benefit the marginal applicant, one whose grades and scores are within range. Having a medical school within a university continues to attract some premed students to that university as undergraduates, as they perceive their chances for admission to their university's medical school as greater than those of outsiders. In any event, even a slight advantage can make a large difference to an individual applicant.

Those medical schools that admitted to weighing more heavily the applicants from more selective institutions did so because these institutions were known to them and the quality of their courses was not in question. More than one medical school admissions director reported that while a student from a more selective school may gain admission with a somewhat lower MCAT score, the applicant from the less selective college will have to have a very strong MCAT score. An admissions committee may be more comfortable taking science grades at their face value when the transcript is from a college or university known to be of high quality; when the institution is not well known, the MCAT, as a standardized measure of competence, will be weighed more heavily. Interviews with admissions directors did not identify any formal weighing system in use.

Acceptance

In 1994, 26,397 men and 18,968 women applied for 16,287 spaces in medical schools, an increase of 18,450 applicants over a 5-year period. As recently as 1991, the ratio of applicants to places was two-to-one. The current acceptance ratio is closer to that of 20 years ago; in 1974, there were 42,624 applicants for 14,763 places, a ratio closer to 3-to-1 (Funkenstein, 1978, p. 26). It is not the case, of course, that each *application* has a likelihood of acceptance that approximates one in two or one in three. Most applicants apply to several (or even 20) schools, and all medical schools receive a quantity of applications many times in excess of the number of students they can accept for their entering classes. The 1994 applicants submitted a total of 561,593 applications (AAMC, 1994b, p. 5).

Many individuals who are not accepted to the next year's class are indeed *qualified for medical school*, if by this is meant that they can do the work required. Their undergraduate academic record is strong and their MCAT scores, average; they are well-rounded, with some leadership experience; they have volunteered or worked for pay in a hospital or laboratory. What makes them *unqualified* is that the admitted applicants ranked higher than they did on some of the quantitative measures and there is a limited number of spaces to be filled in medical schools. One premed student put it this way:

> I thought they [medical schools] would be looking for individuals like me who would be compassionate and believe in preventive medicine. But the AMA seems to be run by those with an old way of thinking. I don't know how or if this will change.

A majority of the first-year premeds thought that cumulative grade-point average and MCAT scores would be the factors weighed most heavily by medical schools when evaluating applications for admission. These are indeed two of the qualifying factors. No other factor, even GPA in science courses, was named by a majority of freshman premeds, although each of these factors was mentioned by one or more individuals: course load or rigor of the academic program, college or university attended, *improvement* in GPA, personality, creativity, confidence level, motivation, compassion, and a memorable one, which expressed faith in the future: "GPA in the junior and senior years." MCAT and cumulative GPA were joined by GPA in science courses as the only admission criteria specified by a majority of premeds in their second year.

By the fourth year, most of the premeds still mentioned only MCAT, cumulative GPA, and science GPA as important qualifications for medical school. As noted earlier, however, admissions directors in medical schools also find merit in the quality of the undergraduate institution, science- and medicine-related employment, health-related community service, extracurricular activities, and the quality of the student's interview with medical school faculty and students. It is particularly surprising that only one in five students who were still interested in medicine attributed importance to the medical school interview.

GENDER AND MEDICINE

The achievements of women have been limited by structural and cultural constraints. Structural constraints include blocked entrance to an occupation (including no or only limited access to the necessary education or training) or blocked mobility within the occupation. Cultural constraints include the prevailing views of what occupations and degrees of participation in careers are appropriate for different categories of people in the society. Cultural constraints are operating when a category of children is socialized "to want or not to want to achieve certain goals and they act on the basis of this socialization" (Cole, 1986, p. 550). In a historical study of acceptance rates of women and men to medical schools, Cole found that in schools that accepted women at all there was "virtually no difference in the acceptance rates of men and women" between 1930 and 1984 (p. 554). Although some medical schools did not accept women until the middle of the present century, all medical schools were admitting women well before the end of that period. So, by this measure, structural constraints on women entering medical school had been removed. Yet reports of medical school as a male-dominated-and-influenced institution are still heard. The leadership in medical schools is predominantly male and the culture within the institution, by some accounts, still is male (Gose, 1995b, p. A49). While the rates of acceptance of women to medical school point to a lessening of the structural constraints of an earlier time, cultural constraints remain.

McLure and Piel (1978) collected data from college-bound high school senior girls in an attempt to learn about the barriers they perceived to launching careers in scientific fields. The four barriers cited most often were the difficulty, length, and expense of a scientific career; the concern about combining family with career demands; the lack of information regarding science careers; and the lack of encouragement from teachers and counselors. On the other side of the issue, these young women listed encouragement from family and changing career opportunities for women as conditions that operate to encourage women to pursue scientific careers.

The study of gender differences in occupational choice over time has shown the effects of the strong and visible women's movement in the United States, especially since the start of the 1970s. The consciousness-raising begun by the second wave of this movement during the 1960s, combined with anti-discrimination legislation at state and federal levels, has resulted in a decrease in overt discrimination, with women entering in growing numbers what once were male-dominated occupations. Attitudes, too, have changed among boys and girls, their parents, and their teachers regarding the occupations that are appropriate for each gender. College students today are less likely to view a career in science as male. As one illustration: 9% of all women entering college in the fall of 1993 reported in Astin's national survey that their career goal was a medical degree, compared with 8% of men (Cage, 1994, p. A29). This is not to say, however, that the experiences of men and women are the same in pursuit of their careers or in the trade-offs they make in other areas of their lives while obtaining the necessary academic and professional credentials. They are not the same. In an extensive review of literature on background characteristics of women in male-dominated occupations, one author noted that women who went on to pursue those occupations were allowed as young children the "opportunity to explore and develop independently." They were not overly restricted in their movements, were granted some independence and the opportunity "to witness a wide range of male and female models" (Lemkau, 1979, p. 228).

Parents who permit their children to explore and learn independently will enable both their sons and daughters to pursue their individual interests later on, with less regard for the perceived gender appropriateness of that interest.

Designations of occupations as inappropriate for women or men, whether made by parents, teachers, counselors, peers, or those practicing within the occupation, have not disappeared but are less likely now to be expressed so straightforwardly. Attributions of appropriateness may relate to the dominance of men or women in the occupation, or to the tasks performed on the job. Even when barriers are being crossed, resistance within the occupation may take a long time to overcome and expectations a long time to change. A woman in an undergraduate engineering program reported (in a personal communication to me) that when her class was scheduled to visit a construction site, the men in the class dressed down for the trip, wearing jeans and athletic shoes. The women, future engineers, too, were told by the course instructor to wear skirts or dresses and heels to the site. It was clear to this woman that the men and women in the class were not expected to participate in the same way in this field experience, although all expected to be engineers within a few years. Gender appropriateness may also relate to the relationship between the occupation and its demands and the competing demands of future nonoccupational roles. Women, to a greater degree than men, even among the premed students followed in this study, have factored in the effects of a particular occupational choice on personal relationships and family roles. This picture of *male* and *female* experience is painted with a broad brush; some individual men and women will have experiences more similar to one another than different.

The structure of the employment market, even for physicians, is such that new entrants to the profession are unlikely to be able to effect major changes in the short run, even if they want to do so. The very process of competing with so many high-achieving peers is likely to make the accepted medical student happy just to be *in*. While some women medical students draw attention to the male or even sexist climate of some medical schools (Gose, 1995b), an open question is how medicine will change in the long run as a result of the influx of women in greater numbers than ever before.

SUPPLY ISSUES

How many doctors is enough? What constitutes oversupply and shortage? The prospective medical student shares with much of the general population an incredulous reaction when it is suggested that there are too many doctors.

Why, then, must an individual often make an appointment far in advance to see a doctor and even then often sees the doctor, especially a specialist, for only a very brief time? Yet there are recommendations from health-policy experts for cutting the number of students admitted to medical schools (Gose, 1995a). This is not the first wave of such recommendations, however. As far back as 1932 the Commission on Medical Education, financed largely by the AMA, "suggested that medical colleges be required to reduce the number of graduates 25% each year until a ratio of one Doctor to 2,000 of the population is reached" (Rayack, 1967, p. 74).

> The report argued, an oversupply [of physicians] is likely to introduce excessive economic competition, the performance of unnecessary services, an elevated total cost of medical care, and conditions in the medical profession which will not encourage students of superior ability and character to enter the profession. (p. 73)

Three factors that contribute to the definition of the physician supply as scarcity or surfeit are expectations, finances, and alternatives. With the advances in medical technology and the availability of Medicare and Medicaid, we have come to expect that all of our illnesses and injuries will be treated successfully. With health insurance programs, we have come to attend less to the issue of cost. Yet expensive medical technology is difficult for hospitals to fund. Some very sophisticated equipment, which will be used infrequently at individual hospitals before it is out-of-date, can be utilized more frequently at regional medical centers that can specialize in this sort of procedure. This degree of centralization is inconvenient for patients, however, as they must travel to obtain the treatment and may have to wait longer for it. It is disadvantageous, too, to an individual medical student who chooses one of the specialties for which fewer placements will be available.

As new medical technology becomes available, specialists trained to use the technology want it to be available in their institutions. Hospitals competing for patients recognize the advantage of being state-of-the-art. Patients, however, have access only to those procedures that their insurance companies will pay for, while expecting that whatever is available *out there* that could benefit them should be accessible. Salaries will remain high for those doctors who do receive specialty training and who are at these prestigious regional medical centers keeping up-to-date on the latest technology. While from the patient's point of view the *need* for this specialty is high—that is, the patient values the convenience of having the service available locally if the insurance company will pay for it—the need as perceived by the medical administrators is low and can be met best by delivering medical care in a more centralized way.

The third factor is alternatives. Nurses, therapists, and other highly trained professionals in the health field are delivering services that once were provided only by doctors. While the patient may want to have a lengthy conversation with a doctor about his or her condition and have the doctor perform all services, such is no longer the norm. The days of doctors making home visits, giving shots, and measuring blood pressure are gone. Until the 1950s, doctors routinely made house calls. When they stopped making such calls, the reaction from older patients in particular was one of disbelief: How could a sick person be expected to travel to the doctor? Yet that quickly became the expectation, and the ratio of doctors to the total population that is *needed* changed significantly as more and more doctors practiced only in their offices and in affiliated hospitals. Rayack (1967), looking only at the 20-year period from 1939 to 1959, noted that the number of physicians increased 35%, in comparison, for example, with a 626% increase in physical therapists and a 77% increase in the number of professional nurses.

Some students who see their chances for acceptance to an allopathic medical school as far from certain choose to apply to schools of osteopathic medicine. Osteopathy as developed by its originator, Andrew Taylor Still, is described as "a system of manipulation intended to realign the abnormalities [osteopathic lesions] . . . in and about the joints of the musculoskeletal system, particularly in the spinal column" (Rayack, 1967, p. 241). More recently, osteopathy has developed in ways that are often indistinguishable from allopathic medicine, and the curricula for students pursuing doctor of osteopathy (DO) and MD programs are quite similar. A number of the students in our study who applied to DO programs did so not so much because they viewed osteopathy as a preferred way to practice medicine, but because they saw the differences as relatively minor. Furthermore, admission to DO programs was still less competitive than to MD programs. Their desire to practice medicine was too strong to be deterred by the difference in prestige between the two different types of medicine.

There also has been an increase in interest in homeopathic practices in recent years. While homeopathy was strong in the United States early in this century, the number of practitioners had declined significantly; but it is now on the rise again. One might suspect that it is the personal attention that the individual patient receives from the homeopathic practitioner, in comparison with the allopathic doctor in the HMO, that explains some of this increase.

PREMED BIOGRAPHIES: BACKGROUND AND PRE-COLLEGE EXPERIENCE

There is some danger in moving from the observation that medical schools are looking among the applicants for those who have mastered the academic challenges posed by an undergraduate premed program to the conclusion that there is a *premed type*. To dispel this notion, 10 of the premed study participants will be profiled throughout the book. Their personal characteristics, family backgrounds, and pre-college academic experiences will be introduced here. These 10 premed students I have named Amy, Ben, Charles, Chris, Dan, Emily, Lynn, Marsha, Michael, and Nora.

Amy is white, the oldest child in her family. She lived with her parents, both of whom were employed. Her mother has a college degree and her father, a graduate professional degree. Amy attended a public high school, where she decided that she wanted to be a doctor. She took advanced placement (AP) biology, chemistry, and calculus courses. Her favorite subject was mathematics, and her favorite course was calculus. While her SAT scores were in the mid 1400s (all scores converted to the recentered SAT scale), her grades in math and science courses were mostly Bs.

Ben is white, the older of two children, and lived with both parents. They were employed; his father has a college degree. While attending a private all-male high school, Ben took no science beyond the introductory courses in biology, chemistry, and physics, nor did he take calculus. Physics was his favorite course. While he had developed his interest in medicine as a young child and might have taken advanced courses in science, they were not offered at his high school. His grades across subjects were mostly A and A–; his SAT scores, too, were high, at 1400.

Charles is African American, an only child. He lived with his parents, who were employed. He attended public high school, where he took no extra science courses and did not take calculus, but earned mostly As in the science and math courses he took. Charles decided on medicine in his senior year, while he was enrolled in a physics course. His SAT scores were just over 1100.

Chris is white, the younger of two children. He attended a coed private high school. His mother has a graduate professional degree and was employed; his father is deceased. Chris decided on medicine when he was a child. He took a second year of biology, his favorite subject, and his course in anatomy was his favorite. He liked the course because the teacher made the material interesting. He earned mostly Bs in his science and math courses, and he scored 1300 on the SAT.

Dan is white, the younger of two children. He lived with his parents, both of whom were employed. His mother has a college degree. Dan attended a public high school, where he took no extra science courses and no calculus. With only one exception, he earned As in all of his math and science courses. His favorite subject was biology, and he decided on medicine early in high school. His SAT scores were 1200.

Emily is white, a middle child, who lived with her parents. Her father was employed; both of her parents have graduate professional degrees. She made her initial choice of medicine as a young child. Emily took no extra science courses at the public high school that she attended, but she did take calculus. Unlike a majority of premeds in the study, her favorite subject was other than math or science. Her science grades were good, better than her math grades, and she scored above 1150 on the SAT.

Lynn is Asian American, the older of two children. She lived with both parents, who were employed. Her father has a college degree. At her public school, Lynn took AP biology and AP calculus. Although she had chosen medicine as a child, both her favorite course and her favorite subject were other than math and science. A history course was her favorite because the teacher taught her how to write good essays. She earned mostly As and her SAT scores exceeded 1400.

Marsha is white, a middle child, living with both parents. Her father has a college degree and was employed. Marsha decided on medicine when she was in junior high but took no extra science courses in an honors curriculum in her public high school. She did take calculus, which she later described as her favorite course, although math was not her favorite subject. She said that her calculus teacher was "wonderful" and "could pull out from students things they didn't think they knew." She earned As and one B in her math and science courses and scored 1450 on the SAT.

Michael is white, the older of two children. He lived with his parents, both of whom were employed. His father has a college degree. At an all-male private high school, Michael took calculus, but no extra science courses, in an honors curriculum. Mathematics was his favorite subject, but he earned As in all his science courses as well as his math courses. He decided on medicine while in high school, having been impressed by some doctors whom he had met. His SAT score exceeded 1300.

Nora is African American, the younger of two children. She lived with her parents, both of whom were employed. Her father has a graduate professional degree. She attended public high school, where she was enrolled in an honors math curriculum, in which she earned A– grades. Nora took AP courses in calculus and in chemistry. Her SAT score was 1250. Chemistry was her favorite subject, but AP calculus was her favorite course: "The teacher was very good. I had not thought I would do well, but I did, and gained confidence." She decided on medicine while in high school.

SEVEN OF THESE students were graduates of public high schools and the remaining three of private high schools. They came into this premed program with unequal levels of science preparation, and only one had completed more than one year of chemistry before starting college. In succeeding chapters, we will see how they fared in their premed program.

Chapter 3

CHOOSING MEDICINE

"Being the doctor would be nice." (a student reporting on her observation of doctors in a hospital setting)

The initial choice of an occupation is not in any sense a commitment, but it does set in motion a sequence of actions that can build to a commitment. Students choosing law, in contrast to those choosing medicine, need not take any action until the junior or senior year in college, when they take the standardized admission test for law school. Medicine requires early action, in the selection of high school and college courses. And performance in these courses provides ongoing opportunity to reevaluate the student's initial choice of medicine and science. Success in the next course assumes mastery of the content of the previous course. Success at each stage, especially in mathematics and science, increases confidence in tackling the next stage. Failure, or only limited success, reduces confidence. Bandura (1977) describes this phenomenon as "efficacy expectations," which are influenced by the difficulty of the task attempted, the presence of obstacles, and confidence in the ability to perform the task. Students differ in their expectations for success in premedicine, and expectations influence persistence.

Few occupations captivate children and retain their interest beyond their early fantasy choice and into the period of career exploration and initial preparation as medicine does. Children are exposed to doctors while they are young and impressionable. Half of the students in one early sample had decided on medicine by the age of 13 (Merton, Reader, & Kendall, 1957), although some research has documented that boys decide earlier than girls (Kutner & Brogan, 1980). Astin, reporting on data from a longitudinal study of youth who scored very high on measures of intellectual aptitude, noted that "29% of the boys who had decided to become doctors in the ninth grade still planned on it one year after graduation from high school, while only 9% of the girls had retained these career plans" (quoted in Lopate, 1968, p. 28). Fifty-seven percent of the students participating in my premed study chose medicine as their career prior to the start of high school; an additional 30% selected medicine between the ninth and eleventh grades. There was no difference in the timing of this choice between those whose mother, father, or both, were doctors and those whose parents were in other occupations.

The choice of an occupation, especially a professional occupation, is one of the most significant decisions a person will make. While a growing number of men and women are making the choice more than once, it is seldom easy. Each career choice or change involves some commitment of time (to additional education or training) and of money (the cost of this education and the earnings lost during the training period, as well as debt incurred while not employed). Time devoted to this training is not available for other commitments and pursuits, including family activities and social time with friends. Nor is it a certainty that even a highly motivated person will eventually succeed. Medicine is extreme in these regards. The selection process is competitive, the education required is lengthy and costly, and the work is demanding, with its unscheduled hours and the stress of knowing that mistakes can have serious consequences. In medicine, the practitioner's primary loyalty is to medicine—not to family, friends, community, or other interests. It is a *greedy* occupation (Coser, 1974). Even the status of *premed* has meaning, for outsiders as well as for participants, of a sort that *pre-other occupations* do not share. There are characteristics assumed and an identity shared among participants that differ from those of most other occupational preparation programs.

OCCUPATIONAL CHOICE

Social scientists have long been concerned with studying the ways in which people make major decisions—the prior assumptions they have made and the sort of information they seek to make their choice among alternatives. These theoretical models focus on specific decision opportunities and differ from the developmental models of Ginsberg and others. One model of the choice process has dominated this literature, generating extensive discussion and scholarship, both pro and con. This is the rational model of decision making.

A Prominent Model of Choice

The rational choice model, developed initially by economists, has been applied to a wide range of choices. Its initial applications were to those decision situations where an optimal choice, the highest return on investment, could be identified. The decision maker was assumed to be acting on the basis of self-interest, choosing from among a set of decision alternatives under conditions of risk, where different alternatives carried different levels of risk. The model was later modified for decision situations under conditions of uncertainty, where the probabilities of the alternative outcomes could not be specified in advance because there was too much contingency or too little information. Under these conditions no option could be labeled *best*, only some as better than others, to reach a specified goal. The decision maker, acting on the basis of self-interest, with some knowledge of a range of choice alternatives and equipped with a value system that permits some ranking of alternatives, selects an alternative that is preferred to the other options in some way(s). Simon (1957) described the process of behaving rationally within real constraints as *bounded rationality*. Decision makers (including college students making career decisions) often proceed in an *intendedly rational* way (March, 1994), acting *as if* their actions were directly linked to known consequences. Persons making what they expect to be long-term career choices often proceed as if they were acting rationally. They attempt at certain points to relate perceived options to their personal goals, and they evaluate their progress toward these goals with whatever information is available to them. At least they are likely to recall having acted in that way.

Weick (1995) argued that decision makers understand and make sense of a decision only by looking back and reconstructing the decision process, which often appears to have been more systematic and inevitable than it actually was. Rationality connotes planning, and persons place value on having planned the important decisions in their lives. For this reason, they may take credit for such planning even when it did not take place. The interviews in this study encouraged participants to reflect on the previous year(s) and may have resulted in their recollection of decisions as highly planned and rational. The structured premed curriculum, too, with sequenced courses, reinforces the notion of rationality.

Deciding what is valued is an early and important aspect of the choice process. Establishing what is good or desirable enables a person to begin evaluating possible ways of maximizing these values. Wealth, intellectual challenge, autonomy, service to others, and social recognition are found in varying quantities and in different combinations across occupations. These quantities and combinations can vary also within an occupation over time, complicating the decision process. For example, a physician has less autonomy now than she or he once had. Doctors today and in the near future are more likely to be working in group practices or in HMOs, where their own professional goals and priorities will not always prevail. The rewards of income, service, recognition, and challenge remain strong, however, in comparison with other occupations.

A major limitation of a rational model when applied to the long-term process of occupational choice is that it assumes self-interest throughout the process, a condition that will not be met in choosing a career. As Etzioni (1992) noted, the rational model excludes "affective involvements" (p. 97), aspects of life that are very significant in the decision to pursue medicine (or not). Personal relationships with parents, peers, and intimates may figure prominently in the choice of a career. People make their life decisions, including those concerning a career, within a social context, influenced in part by the preferences and interests of family members and friends. Since nearly all premed students place high value on service to others, their selection of medicine would seem not to be self-interested, again violating an assumption of rationality. From another perspective, however, self-interest is not necessarily ruled out. Unlike many other occupational choices, persons preparing for medicine do not have to choose altruism over income; they can have both. With the exception of doctors practicing in poor inner-city communities, in disadvantaged rural areas, and with international relief efforts, doctors whose primary or sole motivation for the study of medicine is to alleviate suffering do not necessarily earn less. Nor do they receive less recognition for their efforts than those who entered medicine with high earnings as a prominent motivation.

There are many specific decisions en route for the premed and even the pre-premed student: to stay in or drop a course, to register for the next course, to volunteer in a hospital or join an emergency medical team, to take the MCAT. Data for this study were collected at three major decision points: at the close of each of the first two years in college, when students must decide whether or not to register for premed courses next year, and early in the fourth year, when they decide whether or not to complete the process of applying to medical schools. Premed students make their decisions about curriculum and career with the knowledge that there are a limited number of opportunities for a much larger number of opportunity seekers. This competition constrains rational decision making, too. Some premeds do not perceive that they are making decisions as they go along, because they decided at an earlier time to *stick it out*, even when their performance was weaker than that of the competition. Yet they are still making choices.

Having selected medicine as a goal and having made decisions that increased commitment to the goal, the premeds found new attractions to staying in the program. Once identified as premed, some perceived *quitting* to carry negative connotations. More positively, they were part of a cohort of premed students going through the same experience. People can be attracted to groups because they are attracted to a task the group is working on, because they value the opportunity to associate with the other members, or because they like the prestige of the group. As one premed said, "Nonpremed people are impressed that I am in the premed program." Most premeds began because of their attraction to the work that doctors do, yet over time they may be sustained by the association with other premeds, because of friendships already made, or because pursuit of this curriculum is regarded by other students as requiring intellect and dedication.

Stages in the Choice Process

Some of the early theory and empirical research on occupational choice described this developmental process as consisting of a series of identifiable stages. Ginsberg, Ginsberg, Axelrod, and Herma (1951) labeled the stages the fantasy, tentative, and realistic periods. The fantasy stage is the earliest, where the child "chooses" an occupation, making a very preliminary choice without consideration of ability or other constraints. As noted earlier, over half of the students in this study made their initial selection of medicine as their career at a young age:

> I've always wanted to be a doctor.

> It was never a decision for me; it was a childhood dream.

> I've wanted to be a doctor since I was 7 years old.

> I have wanted to be a doctor since I was 3 years old.

The tentative stage is subdivided into four substages: interest, capacity, value, and transition (Ginsberg et al., 1951). A child starts with a set of interests and continues to narrow the focus to those that are linked with abilities already evident. The boy or girl who attends a performance of a children's symphony and decides to become a concert musician has expressed a tentative interest. After several months of music lessons, that child's capacity can be measured. Lacking the necessary combination of talent and discipline, the child will not sustain the dream of becoming a musician in a symphony orchestra. The (older) child begins to recognize the different values of a range of occupations. In the transition from tentative exploration to reality testing, the individual tests the chosen occupation—in a college curriculum, with vocational training, employment, or community service. Testing continues until these experiences crystallize a career choice, which the individual continues to develop with advanced or specialized training. Since a majority of the premeds made their fantasy occupational choice early in childhood and their tentative occupational choice early in high school, their capacity was tested throughout high school and college. Data on premeds nationally showed that most decided while in high school that they wanted to study medicine (AAMC, 1989).

The tentative choice of medicine was stimulated by success in science, encouragement received from others, and identification with a respected person in medicine. These comments by the premeds indicate influence during the decision-making process:

> In high school, biology was my best subject.

> Medicine was always an option; both of my parents are doctors.

> My mother is a nurse.

> To capitalize on my success in science.

> My parents have told me since I was young [that I should be a doctor].

Some students could even point to a catalytic event that resulted in their selecting a medical career:

> I had a relative with cancer in the summer before my junior year of high school.

> During the summer after my junior year of high school I was working as a lifeguard, and a girl jumped off the board and broke her leg.

> …as the result of some childhood injuries.

In a study of individuals taking the MCAT in 1992 and 1993, participants who chose medicine as their profession before or during high school (29% and 31% of boys, and 34% and 37% of girls) gave as the most important influence on their decision to pursue medicine the influence of one or both parents, work or other related experience, or an illness or accident (AAMC, 1994a, p. 81).

The early work on occupational choice, while providing some concepts for understanding the developmental process, excluded the experience of girls and women. When women were mentioned, it was usually in a discussion of their not being as free as men to make occupational choices but rather having to fit any occupational activity around a husband and children. The assumption that marriage and children will happen for every woman and will define her primary identity from that point on is still often implicit. Consequently, this logic runs, it is difficult for a woman to plan for any full-time career.

Gender stereotyping has diminished over time, however, and the vocational preference tests frequently used by career and guidance counselors have been revised to be more gender-neutral. Yet the old models of occupational selection have held their ground because their focus on developmental stages is intuitively appealing. One of these models is employed here as a heuristic device, as it seems generally to describe the experience of women as well as men in our study. Research (Kerr & Maresh, 1994) has documented that the interests and career aspirations of gifted girls are more similar to those of gifted boys than of other girls. While it is not the case that all or even most premed students are gifted, they tend to be high achievers, and in an institution with high admission standards, we would expect less gender difference than among the larger population of college students.

The research by Ginsberg et al. (1951) was conducted with college-bound boys. Included, too, was a very small sample of 10 women students from Barnard College, a highly selective women's college. These women were not observed or interviewed as children, so there is no first-hand information available on the early stages of their career development. However, they did recall their aspirations as children. According to the authors, "the recollections . . . of their vocational behavior during the early stages of the Tentative period correspond closely to the behavior observed in the interviews with boys 11 to 15" (Walsh & Osipow, 1994, p. 78).

The men and women in our study were privileged with respect to education and parental attention. Some also enjoyed economic and cultural advantages. To the extent that such advantages diminish gender differences in aspirations, expectations, and opportunities, the premed women should experience the four stages similarly to men. Some of the premeds expressed the concept of progression through stages this way:

> College is a personal journey. You no longer are doing things for your parents but are discovering your own interests.

> Last year I was doing it for Dad; now I'm doing it for me.

> I realize that I need not plan so far ahead. I do not think of myself as a cardiovascular surgeon [now]; I'm taking it one step at a time.

> Until my sophomore year [in college] I said, "I want to be a doctor" without understanding what that meant. Then I became more mature and questioned whether being a doctor was what I wanted. After thinking seriously about it, I decided "yes," because I want to help people.

While in high school, the (pre-)premeds discussed their career plans with family members, teachers, and counselors and took the college preparatory science and mathematics courses that serve as preparation for college-level study of these subjects. Many students also volunteered in hospitals, where they observed the practice of medicine and talked with doctors they knew. They continued their exploration of a medical career by taking general chemistry in the first year of college, joining the premed society, and continuing community service related to health care. They persisted unless they met an overwhelming obstacle, encountered a more attractive career alternative, or simply had too little reward for the effort: "I would like medicine as a career, but the coursework is preventing me from this." This student went on to say that although she studied very little in high school, she had been at the top of her class. High school experience did not always prepare the premeds for the rigors of the college program.

What help do students receive in their high schools for course and career choices? The counselor does not emerge as a key figure in the experience of adolescents in some larger high schools, where there are so many students to be seen that the counselor cannot spend a great deal of time one-on-one with anyone. This may be a reason why a number of students reported that they received more support from their teachers for continuing with advanced math and science courses and pursuing a career in medicine than from counselors. When asked about the source of their information on premed and medicine programs before entering college, a majority said that their primary source was family members or family friends. A minority reported that their information came from their high school teachers or counselors. Some premeds' comments suggested that they faulted their counselors, not for providing inaccurate information but for failing to impress on them the rigors of the college premed program. The counselors should not be faulted for this. Many students who excelled during high school were unable to imagine not doing as well in college. For those students, any cautions expressed by the counselor would have fallen on deaf ears: "They didn't tell me that you have to really want it in order to succeed." Another student reported an unconventional approach used by a counselor: "My high school counselor gave me course information and yelled at me when I did badly."

HIGH SCHOOL ACADEMIC PROGRAM AND SUPPORTING BEHAVIOR

Some students enter college premed programs better prepared than their peers. While a strong foundation in math and science is one aspect of that preparation, so, too, is the discipline developed from good study habits and putting academics first. School activities, unstructured time with friends, and, for many students, employment, all compete for the high school student's time, and establishing priorities with academics first can be difficult.

Course of Study

In order to succeed in a premed program, any student must enter college having completed at least one year each of biology, chemistry, and physics in high school. Many of the participants in this study took additional science as well as calculus. All the students in the study had completed at least one year of biology in high school; over half had taken a second year. Only one student had not taken any chemistry in high school, and one in six had taken 2 years of chemistry. Most students also took a physics course; a second year of physics is seldom offered, except in those high schools concentrating in mathematics and science. Fifty students, nearly a third of my sample, had taken more than one science course in a year while in high school. Many students in college are still anxious about doubling up on science courses with laboratories, yet it is something that medical schools will expect to find when evaluating an applicant's college transcript. Two laboratory science courses taken simultaneously will be a fact of life in medical school. Students who have had this sort of course load in high school will be better prepared for their future course schedules.

For the participants in this study, grades in their high school biology courses were good overall, yet there was some variation in the distribution. The grade earned most often in Biology I by these premeds was A, but four students earned C or lower grades in this course and 18 others B– to C+. The distributions of grades in chemistry and physics were similar, with A the grade received most often. A strong background in mathematics contributes to success in college-level science. Nearly half of the premeds had completed Algebra I prior to starting high school; the rest took the course in ninth grade. Most followed the college preparatory track in mathematics from Algebra I to geometry and Algebra II, to trigonometry/pre-calculus. The differentiation began only with Calculus I, usually in the twelfth grade. Calculus is not a required course in most college preparatory curricula, although it may be (strongly) recommended by teachers or counselors for students who plan to continue in science and mathematics. Nearly half of the premeds took a calculus course while in high school, and most of them earned A or B grades. Some planned to continue that course sequence in college with a second calculus course, to satisfy the admission requirements of some medical schools. Since two-thirds of our students had earned grades of B or higher in trigonometry, most should have been able to succeed in calculus.

There is a penalty levied on students who do not progress through the basic 4-year college preparatory math curriculum in high school (through pre-calculus), which does not apply to those who do not complete the full range of science courses. A student can take a science course at the college level without having studied the subject in high school, but many colleges do not offer *pre*-calculus courses. Students lacking adequate preparation in high school mathematics will find that certain programs or majors are inaccessible without first completing this remedial work, which may not be offered by their college. Biology was the high school subject identified most often as the favorite; indeed, it was a liking for biology that steered many of these students toward medicine. Overall, this population of premed students demonstrated early success in science and math, keeping open a range of academic and career options, whether they remained premed or not.

Most of these premed students (90%) said that when they entered college, their information about the premed program was at least *pretty accurate*. While 65% of them said that their information in high school about what was to follow in college had no effect on their choice of high school courses, the remainder took more math and science courses than they would have taken otherwise. Some of the students for whom the information had no effect on their high school curriculum had no choice among courses; they were taking the most rigorous (science) curriculum offered at their school.

Activities Outside the Classroom

While the link between a strong academic foundation in high school and later achievement in college is obvious, the relationship between extracurricular activities and other free-time pursuits and achievement and persistence in a college premed program may be less evident. In grade 9, these future premeds spent an average of 6 to 10 hours per week in extracurricular activities. By the junior and senior years, when students were more likely to be employed part-time, they were *also* spending 11 to 15 hours in extracurricular activities. They all spent some time on such activities as a high school senior, and some reported devoting more than 30 hours a week to extracurricular activities. While it would not be possible to cover the wide range of these activities, some were listed frequently: varsity athletics, student government, and community service. Commitment to an activity over time while still in high school can benefit a student once in college. Commitment entails enduring the bad with the good, as well as postponing gratification now in anticipation of future rewards. These aspects of commitment also characterize successful progress through premedical and medical education. The measure of commitment used in this study combined hours per week spent in an activity with the number of years of involvement. Slightly over half of the participants exhibited commitment at the level of 5 or more hours per week in an activity over 4 years, receiving the highest score on the commitment scale.

Nearly two-thirds of those interviewed spent 1 to 5 hours per week on household chores while in high school; only one in four students spent more time. Nearly a third of the premeds were responsible for the care of younger siblings or other family members, often in addition to their household chores. These data are not out of line with previous research findings (White & Brinkerhoff, 1981a, 1981b), which show that while gender and number of children, family status (one or two parent), parents' employment, and urban/rural location can impact on the household chores that children are expected to do, most families require that some of this work be assumed by the children. The stated purpose is to instill a sense of responsibility and build their character (White & Brinkerhoff, 1981a). As these children get older and have the opportunity to enroll in demanding academic programs that require more time to complete assignments out of class, they may be conflicted if they have a great deal of work to do at home, including caring for younger siblings, and also must find sufficient uninterrupted time for study and homework. While most of our students were not so obligated, some did have extensive responsibility at home, including a few who worked as reserve labor in the family business, expected to fill in whenever they were needed.

Using data from a national survey, Marsh (1991) looked at the effects of employment on high school students. Specifically, he concluded that "total hours worked unfavorably affected . . . standardized test scores . . . [and] the selection of science courses," among a number of other outcomes (p. 179). These effects were noted after accounting for the influence of other, especially background, variables. While high school employment takes time away from other activities, including studying, employment sometimes is necessary for students who must supplement a low family income or contribute significantly to their future college expenses. This was less common in the premed sample, where only 14% of students employed during the year in high school worked to pay for college expenses. Extracurricular activities, in contrast to employment, are on the school calendar and are designed in part to develop skills that complement the curriculum. Employment can make demands of time or energy that are outside the control of the school and the individual employee. Students who work during high school because they feel they have to may put their employment first and make accommodations to their study schedule. They will have a difficult time meeting the demands of a rigorous curriculum. Less than one-quarter of the premeds were employed part-time in grades 9 or 10; by grade 11, however, nearly half were employed. By the senior year, part-time employment was the norm (51%), with students working anywhere from 2 to 40 hours per week, 15 on average. When asked why they were employed, their most frequent answer (from 53%) was "to earn spending money."

Other research (Steinberg, Fegley, & Dornbusch, 1993) has shown that the negative impact of employment on school performance occurs for those high school students employed more than 20 hours a week. That research showed that students working long hours may maintain their grades by taking easier courses or those with less demanding teachers. Our premeds took a full college preparatory curriculum in high school, and their high school GPAs were recalculated by the university admission office, eliminating any peripheral or *fluff* courses. Yet a small number of them had been employed 20 or more hours a week, with no obvious impact on later persistence in the premed program.

Social Influences

Everyone takes cues from others, paying particular attention to the responses and evaluations of persons they like, respect, or want to be like. Adolescence is a time of great change—physical, emotional, psychological—and conformity is a way of going through these changes with less scrutiny. In peer groups where academic success is not valued or even accepted, it is difficult for adolescents to choose success in school while sacrificing acceptance by peers. The term *reference group* was used first by Herbert Hyman in 1942 "to denote a group in which an individual is motivated to gain or maintain acceptance" (Hyman, 1968, p. 78). There are normative and comparison reference groups. The former, like family or church, provide standards for behavior (norms), teaching what is right and wrong. The comparison group, on the other hand, provides a basis for a comparative evaluation of performance. As one illustration, premed students in a required science class use the members of the class as a comparative reference group in order to evaluate their own performance on a test. While each test presents an opportunity for students to demonstrate their knowledge or lack of same of the subject matter, testing also is an opportunity to measure achievement in comparison with others in the class.

Sometimes the normative and comparison functions may be performed by a single group (Hyman, 1968). For many adolescents, this is the peer group, which can serve as the source of behavior standards and the basis for comparison. Any student who has completed even a portion of the premed science curriculum can claim premed as a reference group. At many universities, including the one where this study was conducted, there is no formal check on who is in or out of the program until it is time to submit applications to medical schools. Consequently, even weaker students can be *premed*.

One area of adolescent life strongly influenced by peers is dating. No questions asked in any of the interviews produced greater discomfort than those about high school dating. Dating, as a free-time activity, competes with other interests and responsibilities, including studying, for the limited time available. There are norms in the adolescent peer group about dating frequency, and while the students interviewed were not asked about those norms, we were sure without asking that they existed. When people violate norms, they are uncomfortable. Students who dated infrequently or not at all were more uncomfortable than other respondents answering questions on dating. In the ninth grade, two-thirds of the future premed students did not date at all or did not date more often than once a month. Nearly half dated less than once a month or not at all while in tenth grade. In grade 11 the profile began to change, perhaps related to students' driving by this time. In that year, 75% of students were dating at least once a month, and more than half that number at least once a week. In the senior year, the norm for this student population was dating at least once a week, but a quarter dated less often than once a month or did not date at all when they were high school seniors.

Support for Learning

When learning difficult subject matter, it is easy to get frustrated and give up in the absence of a strong aptitude for the subject and support for continuing. This support may be visible and direct, as when parents and teachers encouraged a student to continue in a math or science sequence. Support may come, too, from friends and family who respect the need for quiet study time. They do not distract the student or tempt her with enjoyable alternatives to studying, nor do they insist that he perform household chores *right now*. The students, too, must develop the discipline necessary to get through the frustrating periods when the learning is slow and the content particularly difficult to master. A small minority of students will not find even the most advanced curriculum difficult, and they may progress with relatively little effort. For the majority, however, "given a certain amount of talent, hard work does win a good grade—in mathematics and the natural sciences" (Riesman, 1980, p. 23). It is in these disciplines that knowledge is acquired through a more or less linear progression, as a person attempts to move from the basic to the more advanced level.

Parents were described most often (by 36% of the premed students) as having been very actively involved in their sons' and daughters' academic experience—discussing course selection and attending parents' programs at the high school. Another 17% were *uninvolved*. When respondents were asked if their parents encouraged enrollment in math and science courses beyond what was minimally required, the response given most often was *we never discussed this*. While it is possible that students made all course decisions without their parents' counsel, it is more likely that many students did not perceive this to be a decision at all; they simply took whatever math and science courses were available to college-bound students in their high school.

When parents provided support, they did so verbally and by providing home conditions conducive to study—giving the student his or her own room, keeping the house quiet on school nights—and providing such resources as money, time, and transportation for course requirements and other enrichment opportunities.

> [Someone] would bring dinner to my room if I needed to study.
>
> I was exempt from chores at home [when I had to study].
>
> My parents sacrificed their own pleasure for me; they stayed home to help me with homework.

Another student reported that one of her parents undertook a lengthy commute each day after a job change so that she would not have to change schools. These responses underscore the point that commitment to a long-term goal can be reinforced by a climate in which the goal can be pursued without distraction. Other parents used resources as rewards—paying for A grades or threatening to withhold resources if grades were low.

Adolescent activities and attitudes, including motivation for academics, course choices, part-time employment and how those earnings are spent, and plans for the future, are influenced by peers. Spade, Columba, and Vanfossen (1997) noted that what appears to be a personal choice—to take a course or not—is influenced by peers and also by the procedures used by schools to assist students in making choices. The premed respondents provided examples of teachers and counselors who steered them toward advanced science and math courses. Charles provided an example of where such help was crucial. His high school had a vocational as well as an academic track, so it was especially important that he be steered toward the classes needed for a science/premed foundation. Peers, too, provided moderate to strong support, suggesting limited influence of a peer culture that discouraged such pursuits. Some of the premeds received social support from others with similarly high ambitions—either in a defined peer group, such as an honors or TAG (talented and gifted) program, or in a less organized group of friends.

PRECOLLEGE GENDER INFLUENCES

The extensive literature on gender and performance in math and science documents the need to take gender into account in understanding why some bright high school girls who are interested in medicine do not complete the courses necessary to be premed in college. Among the explanations given for these gender differences are several that will be addressed here. These include course enrollments; gender of teacher; identification of science and math subjects and related careers as "male," as well as social support for transcending this cultural barrier; self-confidence; and differential abilities.

Science and Math Enrollment and Achievement

Gender differences have been documented consistently in mathematics and less consistently in science (see Holden, 1987). The difference between boys and girls in mathematical achievement is decreasing, although it has not been eliminated, and research on diverse populations of students has yielded inconsistent conclusions. There is some agreement that this discrepancy develops roughly between grades 7 and 10 (Burke, 1989; Meece, Parsons, Kaczala, Goff, & Futterman, 1982) and is evident by the end of high school (Pallas & Alexander, 1983). There is less agreement on the reasons for the difference. Explanations have focused on course enrollments, gender identification of subject matter, the use of mathematics and physical science outside the classroom, math and science ability, confidence, and gender of teachers. All but one of these explanations emphasize social aspects of learning math and science, that is, the degree to which learning these subjects is influenced by the behaviors of others—parents, peers, and teachers, for example. While much of the literature on gender differences in learning and aptitude has focused on mathematics rather than science, mathematics and physical science share a number of characteristics. In the more advanced high school courses and in college courses, physical science is taught with theory and quantitative concepts, and exams and other assignments require students to perform calculations. Science in college and beyond, like mathematics, is cumulative; the basics must be masterered before moving on.

Boli, Allen, and Payne (1985) noted that the benefits to women students of having had women as math teachers in high school included better grades in a college math course (calculus) during the first year of college and increased retention in calculus and chemistry. More recent data from a national sample of high school students, however, showed that gender of the science teacher was unrelated to the performance of both boys and girls (Burkam, Lee, & Smerdon, 1997).

Benbow and Stanley (1980) concluded from their study of gifted boys and girls that boys more often than girls took calculus while in high school. A study of adolescents who took calculus advanced placement tests in high school showed that while more boys than girls took the AP exam (the AB version, but especially the more advanced BC version), there were *no significant differences* in their scores (Benbow & Stanley, 1982). This finding suggests that while girls were less likely than boys to take the high school course that would prepare them for calculus in college, they performed as well as the boys when they did take the course and test. Taking pre-calculus and even calculus during high school is a more common occurrence now, and a decision that can have attractive payoffs. Enrolling in additional mathematics courses can make a student more attractive to a highly selective college and can result in a higher math SAT score, increasing a student's college options. Pallas and Alexander (1983) found that the difference in math SAT scores between women and men was reduced significantly after controlling for mathematics coursework. They concluded that when women take advanced mathematics courses, "they derive the same benefits" from them as men (p. 178). Eccles (1994) noted that course decisions, like other choice situations, involve weighing alternatives. The choice to take an advanced science or math course is the choice not to take another course. Factors influencing the choice include ability in science or math, attitudes of peers, and the individual's current tentative choice of career. A student who in high school anticipates a career in a nonscience and nontechnical field is likely not to take the advanced math or science courses, regardless of ability.

The *differential coursework* hypothesis—that gender differences in performance in math and science are the result of differential course preparation—receives inconsistent support. Women who apply to the more highly selective colleges and universities, of whom these premeds were examples, are likely to have taken more advanced math and science courses than other women, as these colleges will expect, if not require, this preparation. As one woman premed said: "I took the most difficult subjects for admission to good colleges." Yet DeBoer (1984), in a study of students enrolled in one of these colleges, found that, with the exception of math majors, men took more high school math than women, whether they later majored in science, social science, or the humanities. That the women's grades in the high school math courses they did take were higher, on average, than those of their current male peers in college suggests that enrollment was related to factors other than ability. Men (but not women) are expected to take mathematics even when its immediate usefulness for further study or occupation is not evident. Women are likely to take advanced math when doing so is linked closely to a demonstrated interest in pursuing mathematics or a related field later on. Medicine is such a field.

Women in the premed sample were somewhat *more* likely than men to have completed Algebra I prior to the ninth grade. Their next opportunity to choose a math course (or choose not to take math) came with calculus. Men were *less* likely than women (44% to 62%) to have taken a calculus course while in high school. The women premeds who took calculus in high school had earned slightly higher grades than men in trigonometry/pre-calculus, the previous math course, although the difference was not significant. Past performance has been shown to be a weaker predictor of future math course enrollment among men than among women (DeBoer, 1984). Women who had earned lower than a B grade were less likely than men with the same grades to take the calculus course. However, the women who did take calculus in high school earned higher grades in that course than premed men. Aspiring premed students of both genders take biology and chemistry in high school, and a large majority take physics. Women in this sample were more likely than men to have taken a second course in biology (one or two semesters) in high school. As high school students, these women premeds outperformed the men in Biology I, accounting for part of the gender difference in enrollment in Biology II. These data support the notion that women will advance in mathematics and science when their past performance gives them reason to believe they will be successful.

The difference in achievement between men and women in high school chemistry was more surprising: 86% of women but only 68% of men earned B or better grades. Higher achievement by women was also demonstrated in physics, where 87% of women and 72% of men earned B or better grades, with similar percentages of men and women enrolling in this course. This was somewhat surprising, given the large literature that demonstrates a gender gap in high school performance between female-identified and male-identified subjects.

Perhaps these women and men attended different sorts of high schools. More specifically, were women more likely than men to have attended smaller, private schools? The data show that the women were more likely than the men to have attended *public* schools, and the average sizes of their high school classes did not differ. It appears that chemistry is more gender-neutral than has been acknowledged; neither boys nor girls are able to spend significant out-of-class hours working with and hence developing competence with chemicals (Steinkamp & Maehr, 1984). Only the physics grades remain to be explained. Following Kelly's (1987) argument, boys may enroll in physics because it interests them, and girls may be apt to enroll in physics only when they think it will be useful at some later time or when they think they will do well in the subject. While women are less likely to take advanced quantitative courses than men are, they perform somewhat better in the courses they do take (DeBoer, 1984; Pallas & Alexander, 1983).

Gender Identification of Subjects and Roles

If a subject is perceived to be male-identified, whether boys on average show more aptitude for it or not, some girls will turn away from it. As Deaux (1984) noted, gender identification refers to the courses that men and women take and their performance in these subjects, and also to the *perceptions* held by others about *appropriate* mathematics- and science-related behaviors. Parents and others who interact frequently with children can unintentionally reinforce the sense of appropriateness of certain subjects or activities for boys and their inappropriateness for girls.

If parents buy primarily gender-typed toys for their sons and daughters, and encourage *appropriate* play, this is doubly disadvantageous for the girls. Like the boys, they will have a narrower range of play experience at home. Unlike the boys, however, girls have less opportunity to explore any (nontraditional) interests away from the supervision of their parents. Older children can contribute to the gender-typing of activities for a younger child. As one of the premed students reported: "I grew up with Barbies. My [older] sisters prevented my parents from getting me race cars and other toys I wanted."

Teachers, too, can reinforce the perception that a subject is more appropriate for one gender than another—in deciding which students to call on in class, in responding (or not) to a student's question or answer, in determining which students to recommend for higher-level or AP courses in the subject.

Research has shown a relationship between skills developed and knowledge acquired in play activities and an understanding of math and science. Leggos and Tinkertoys can help to develop spatial skills in children, while chemistry sets, microscopes, and ant farms, among others, increase the child's familiarity with the subject matter of science. The study participants were asked if their parents bought science and building toys for them when they were younger. While it had been several years since these young men and women had played with these toys, no one seemed to have forgotten whether they once owned them or not. Forty percent had been given building toys only (45% of the males and 37% of the females), and more had received other science toys, too—49% of the men and 44% of the women. But some had wanted other toys, like one male premed: "I was more interested in sports than in science toys, but my parents bought them all."

Parents may regard math as more useful and important than other subjects for their sons than for their daughters (Eccles & Jacobs, 1986; Parsons, Adler, & Kaczala, 1982). They may also exhibit a gender difference in their own experience with mathematics, with fathers more likely than mothers to say that they were good in math. While these parental views do not always have a strong influence on their children's expectations for their own success in math (Parsons et al., 1982), it is likely that they contribute to a household climate stressing the gender appropriateness of specific abilities and tasks. When parents let their children know they think math is difficult for them (the children) or communicate that they (the parents) are not good in math, this negative assessment is likely to affect the children's own expectations for success in math, even when they possess the ability to succeed. Parents may hold different perceptions of their sons' and daughters' mathematical abilities even when their actual performance in math is the same (Parsons et al., 1982). The result is that even some girls who are talented in math and science can be deterred from these fields.

Premeds interviewed for my study were unlikely to regard math and sciences as subjects in which men earned higher grades than women. Most of these premed men and women also reported that their parents did not regard mathematics and science as male-identified (or female-identified) subjects.

So many educational programs and occupations require facility with quantitative material that it does a child little good to hear at an early age that she or he is not likely to master this subject. This view may be unique to Americans:

> Americans more than any other people attribute success in mathematics to innate ability rather than to hard work. Students, parents, and teachers the world over, except in the United States, believe that everyone can learn mathematics if only they work at it. (Steen, 1987, p. 302)

The literature on socialization to gender roles has documented the influence of parents' education and mother's occupation. Higher education of both parents contributes to a less restrictive view of gender appropriateness, especially for daughters. While 69% of fathers and 46% of mothers of the premed students had completed college, fathers of sons in the premed program were less likely than the fathers of daughters to have earned a graduate or professional degree. Mothers who had not attended college were more likely to be the mothers of the male students. Mothers of the women premeds and fathers of men and women premeds were most likely to be employed in professional and managerial occupations. Mothers of the men were employed more often in technical and sales occupations. Gender alone tells only part of the story, however. As women in this sample were somewhat more likely than men to be the only or the oldest child in the family, the achievement expectations and advantages that their parents had to bestow may have gone disproportionately to this child.

It may not be physical science per se that is viewed as male-identified but sciences where learning in the classroom can be supplemented by leisure-time activity. Repairing a car, assembling audio equipment, or customizing a computer can increase understanding of physics in particular. As already noted, chemistry differs from physics in this regard; *toys* such as chemistry sets probably are used less than other toys, as parents would require that their children be supervised when *experimenting*. While the premed women performed at a level equal to or better than their male peers in their high school math and science courses, an obvious gender difference was noted on *understanding how machines work and how to fix things*. Women were more likely to report little or virtually no understanding. When the question was last asked of a nationwide sample of college freshmen, in 1977, the finding was that women were far less likely than men (10% versus 37%) to evaluate their mechanical ability as average or above average (Astin, 1978). Hedges and Nowell (1995) performed a meta-analysis on test scores of male and female adolescents and young adults. They noted that the largest sex differences occur in areas not generally taught in school (such as mechanical comprehension). Yet some girls have experience working with mechanical and electrical equipment, as one student told us when asked about science toys she had as a child: "I played a lot with circuit-building kits."

Freedom to Learn

Participants in a retrospective study of 4,000 Ph.D. scientists and engineers said that as children they had learned as much about science from their hobbies as from their school work (Tobias, 1990). Yet boys often are given greater freedom to explore their environment without close supervision, helping them to develop skills and an understanding of how things work (Entwisle, Alexander, & Olson, 1994). Girls, even those who are interested in science, are not given as much opportunity as boys to participate in science activities outside the classroom (Fox, 1974; Handel, 1986; Kahle & Lakes, 1983). Girls, too, are more likely than boys to find that peer groups do not support out-of-class interest in science. There are some encouraging exceptions, however, like the premed woman who said: "I had a high level of interest [in biology]. I read the biology text as someone would read a magazine." Mandelbaum (1981) suggested that girls may be able to with-stand some peer pressure to move away from their achievement goals; if these goals "are tucked away deeply and secured within the self . . . the young girl who first imagines a medical career before adolescence, during

Ginsberg's fantasy choice period, can defend herself against the pressures that come with adolescence" (p. 19).

Persons wishing to advance in math and science must be able to devote concentrated and relatively distraction-free time to study. Studying for a test in an advanced math or science course may require careful reading of the more abstract content two or more times. Students whose other responsibilities—household chores, the care of siblings, or part-time employment—must be attended to on a fixed schedule will find less concentrated time for study. Fennema and Peterson (1985) suggested that persons who wish to master complex subject matter "must participate in autonomous learning behavior" (p. 18), including "working independently on high-level tasks, persisting at such tasks, choosing to do and achieving success at such tasks" (p. 20).

There were no gender differences in this premed population in the average time spent on household chores during high school or on the care of siblings or other persons. Men and women spent 5 hours a week or less on these commitments. Among those who reported having spent 6 or more hours a week, men were more likely to have done chores and women to have taken care of siblings or other family members. Males and females differed most on employment in the senior year of high school, when more women than men were employed. There were no differences in the extent of involvement in extracurricular activities, but there was one pronounced difference in type of activity—varsity athletics, in favor of males. A slight majority of both women and men scored in the highest category on the commitment index, participating 5 hours a week or more in any activity during all 4 years of high school.

When parents discourage risk-taking by their daughters and also expect good grades in school, these daughters will be less likely to take the most difficult courses, especially if the added cost of doing so is disapproval from peers. If mathematics is viewed by parents, peers, counselors, or the girls themselves as less necessary for girls, then risking the grade-point average is not worth it, as there is no corresponding reward for doing so. Even though a particular girl may well outperform boys in her advanced math class if she does take the course, there are many inhibitors to her prior decision to enroll. The success of the premed women in our sample is attributed in part to the support they received from their parents, who provided them sufficient freedom to learn.

"Encouragement from parents . . . has emerged as an important causal factor in girls' decisions to elect advanced mathematics courses in high school" (Meece et al., 1982, p. 331). Ware and Lee (1988) found that women majoring in science were more likely than men majoring in science to have had "parents who were involved in their high school activities" (quoted in Oakes, 1990, p. 198). Women premeds in my study reported higher (42% very actively involved) and also lower (20% uninvolved) levels of parental involvement in their high school academic experience than the men, who described their parents as *somewhat* (28%) or *moderately* (33%) involved. What is being measured here is not the parents' actual degree of involvement but their sons' and daughters' assessments of this involvement. Some parents never discussed math and science course enrollments with their children, but among those parents who did, daughters were more likely than sons to say that their parents provided strong encouragement to continue taking courses in these subjects beyond the minimum required. This, too, is less a measure of parents' interest in math and science, or interest in seeing their children succeed, than it is perceived support for their daughters taking courses often defined as male in their subject matter. There was little evidence of gender-typing among parents, yet when it was reported, it was *male* premeds who were more likely to say that their fathers thought math and science were subjects more appropriate for men than women to study.

Confidence

A factor that can be both cause and consequence of enrollment and performance in math and science courses is the degree of confidence in math and science ability expressed by boys and girls. Studies of college, high school, and junior high school students have shown that males were more confident of their ability to perform successfully in mathematics (Betz & Hackett, 1981; Fennema & Sherman, 1977; Sherman, 1983; Yee & Eccles, 1988), even when the girls' past performance in math was superior to that of the boys (Jacobs, 1991). Girls tend to be conservative in estimating their level of ability, even when they do quite well in the task. It appears, then, that many girls lack confidence more than they lack ability. Lack of confidence does not equate to lack of ability or even to poor performance. Even girls in AP classes can describe themselves as *at the bottom of the class* while their teachers describe the same girls as *among the best* in the class (Casserly, 1980). In Boli and colleagues' (1985) interviews with students at Stanford, only 35% of women compared with 47% of men in the first-year calculus course said they were *well prepared* for the course, yet equivalent proportions (58%) of men and women had taken calculus in high school. On paper, men and women were equally prepared for the course, yet their *perceptions* of their math background were quite different.

Confidence of males in their mathematical ability is grounded in past experience in mathematics and in the expectations for the role that quantitative ability will play in their future. Research has shown that men have been more likely than women to value mathematical ability for its role in their future study or career (Betz & Hackett, 1981; Fennema, 1984; Hilton & Berglund, 1974; Yee & Eccles, 1988). When women are convinced of the future value to them of studying mathematics now, they can overcome a lack of confidence in their math ability. And, as already noted, when women were successful in an earlier course in the subject, they are more likely to take the next course.

The premed women on average reported having received no less support than men from high school peers for pursuing math and science courses, suggesting that these women did not have to trade off peer approval for academic success. Men, however, were more likely to describe peer support as strong (44%) or none (26%), while women said that peer support was moderate (32%) or strong (30%). Nor were counselors biased against women; men and women alike reported strong or moderate support from high school teachers and counselors, with women more likely than men to report having received strong support. It may not be experience out of class that is important in boosting confidence and increasing understanding of math and science, but related experience that makes science more familiar. Students in college chemistry courses, for example, can gain extra familiarity with the subject by doing all of the problems at the end of the chapters. As one premed said: "You have to practice with the material. You must do more than just understand in class; you must do the problems."

Different Abilities

Is there a difference in mathematical aptitude between men and women? One gender difference that has been found consistently is in spatial ability, "skill in representing, transforming, generating, and recalling symbolic, non-linguistic information" (Linn & Petersen, 1985, p. 1482). PSAT and SAT test-takers will recognize this type of test question, which requires the test-takers to mentally manipulate a two-dimensional drawing to produce a three-dimensional object. It may be difficult to believe that such a gender-based difference in aptitude would come into play only at the onset of adolescence, but it is possible that this ability, present in differing degrees in girls and boys, manifests itself first on standardized tests that measure the ability. There is some accumulated evidence that the spatial ability of males, on average, exceeds that of females, although these results do not emerge consistently before high school (Maccoby & Jacklin, 1974; Meece et al., 1982). Harris (1979) noted that "as psychological sex differences go, the differences in spatial ability are fairly large; as few as 20–25% of females may reach the average male score" (p. 135). In 1995, N. L. Friedman reported on a meta-analysis of studies of gender, spatial abilities, and mathematical abilities: while differences in spatial ability exist, they seem to be declining in magnitude. One woman interviewed for my premed study did link spatial ability with success in organic chemistry: "I'm not spatially oriented and the concepts were three-dimensional. I didn't get it."

One explanation for the gender difference in spatial abilities is that girls are less experienced in "spatial problem solving" (Connor, Schackman, & Serbin, 1978, cited in Meece et al., 1982, p. 330). This skill may be learned from playing with toys requiring manipulation or by extensive participation in team sports that require players to envision various configurations of players from two teams as they manipulate a ball. Tracy (1987) noted the contrast between toys such as Leggo blocks, erector sets, and vehicles, toys that "must be manipulated so that they work," and *playing* with the furniture in a doll house. "Although the furniture can be manipulated, the continuation of play is not dependent upon . . . a certain set of arrangements of materials" (p. 127). Video games often assume a high level of spatial ability. Since boys play these games more than girls, the spatial skills that the games help to develop yield further advantage to boys. As Birns and Sternglanz (1983) noted: "When boys' toys change as technology progresses and girls' toys do not, it means that we are still preparing men for careers and women for domestic activities and/or low pay, low preparation jobs" (p. 247). If mechanical and electronic toys continue to be designed, sold, and bought more often for boys than for girls, girls in school will continue to be less comfortable with technology and applications of math and physical science. To the degree that low spatial ability inhibits the learning of mathematics, the gender difference is noteworthy for its consequences. Yet, summarizing research at that time, Fennema (1980) noted that there was no relationship between spatial ability and performance in geometry, where some association might have been expected.

Tracy (1987) proposed a comprehensive explanation for gender differences in math performance, incorporating aspects of the explanations already discussed. As the content of math courses moves from the more concrete to the more abstract, more spatial ability is required to learn concepts. To the extent that students have gained out-of-class experience with spatial tasks and other applications of math- and science-related concepts, they will have less difficulty making the jump to more abstract material than students whose expertise is tied more to learning rules and repeating them in new examples. Making matters more difficult is the fact that the learning of mathematics is cumulative—next week's class material presumes an understanding of what was covered this week. While there are numerous opportunities for a student to become discouraged in the learning of mathematics when the material is especially difficult, there are fewer opportunities to catch up once the teacher and class have moved on. Discouraged students may opt out of the full 4-year college preparatory mathematics curriculum.

Occupational Choice

Occupational aspirations differ for boys and girls as early as the fantasy stage. Siegel (1973) asked a sample of children in the second grade what kind of work they wanted to do when they grew up. The boys "chose almost twice the number of occupations that the girls chose" (p. 16) and, even more surprising, "there was no overlap between those occupations selected by boys and those selected by girls" (p. 17). Even at that early age, children absorb from adults, and from stories and other mass media, that there are different career paths for men and women and that boys have a wider range of choices to match an occupation with their interests. MacKay and Miller found in 1982 that "third and fifth grade boys most frequently chose the occupations of policeman, truck driver, pilot and architect, while girls chose nurse, teacher, and stewardess" (Betz, 1994, p. 13). These two studies are relevant because the children who participated would be close in age today to the participants in my premed study. Even when girls aspire to a nontraditional occupation, they may change their minds during the tentative stage. Marini and Greenberger (1978), reporting on a study of eleventh-grade public school students, noted the diversity of aspirations (the occupation I would like to have) expressed by these girls, in comparison with the narrower range of their expectations (the occupation I expect to have).

Among desired careers for individuals with college and post-baccalaureate education, two broad occupational categories that are male-dominated are those in scientific/technical fields and those that can be described as *high status*, yielding high levels of income and social recognition. Medicine is in both categories. To the degree that girls are able to choose from a wide set of occupations prior to the start of college and also receive parental support for their choice, they will be able to follow the high school curriculum that will best prepare them to pursue this field while in college. Waite and Berryman (1985) found, as did Lemkau (1979), that girls were less likely to choose female-dominated occupations when their mothers were more highly educated or themselves were employed in nontraditional occupations. Until recently, a girl's mother was one of few models for her career expectations. Today, girls and young women have access to women in a wide variety of careers, through school-sponsored career days and internships, through part-time employment, and through other relatives and friends. Consequently, their career choices will be predicted less easily from knowledge of their mother's occupation. While many girls still grow up in households where career ambitions for women are not valued, or live in places where women in high-status professions are not so visible, there has been a change in the national culture, expanding opportunities for girls and women.

Social class has influenced career choice. Funkenstein (1978) studied two groups of physicians: the first entering medical school prior to 1975 and the second entering in 1975. The women in the earlier cohort came from a higher social class than their male peers, on average, with a higher rate of employment among the mothers of female medical students and a higher average level of education. No such differences were found in the later group (p. 76). Because federal loans are now available for professional school study, parents can more easily afford to be supportive of the aspirations of both sons and daughters without having to fully finance a lengthy and costly postgraduate program. More women of modest means, like their male counterparts, began applying to medical school when financial aid became available to them.

INFLUENCE OF RACE

This study was begun with no specific expectations regarding the influence of race on behavior and performance. Students in a premed population in a very selective university are in many ways more alike than different. Yet race, in combination with income and wealth, affects opportunities and outcomes in society and is a factor to be considered. For my study, race was divided into three categories: non-Hispanic whites, Asian Americans, and a third category identified in the medical school admissions process as *underrepresented minorities*, racial groups underrepresented in medical school. Comprising this category are African Americans, Hispanic Americans, and Native Americans. While the AAMC does not regard all Hispanic applicants as underrepresented minorities, the size of this sample did not permit further division of the Hispanic category, so all of the Hispanic premeds were included in this designation. The numerical breakdown is as follows: 104 white, 19 Asian American, and 30 underrepresented minority.

The focus in this chapter is on the pre-college experience and the ensuing impact on first-year college experiences. The three racial groups differed on science enrollment in high school. Asian Americans were the most likely (74%) to have taken additional science courses while in high school, beyond the usual college preparatory curriculum of one year each of biology, chemistry, and physics. Sixty percent of whites and 50% of underrepresented minorities took additional science courses. It is likely that advanced courses were available most often in larger and better-funded high schools, so the degree to which course selection was an individual choice could not be determined. Asian Americans took calculus in high school with greater frequency, too: 79% versus 51% of whites and 41% of premeds from underrepresented minorities. It may have been the case that Asian American students took more science and math in high school because, on average, they made earlier career decisions, with 75% deciding before high school that they wanted to be doctors. In contrast, 57% of whites and of underrepresented minority groups made their career decision that early.

High commitment to an activity (5 or more hours a week for 4 years) was the norm for a majority (58%) of whites and Asian Americans and for 45% of underrepresented minorities. A higher percentage of white students (57%) than of underrepresented minorities (48%) or Asian Americans (38%) was employed during high school. None of the employed Asian Americans, compared with 20% of the whites, and 43% of underrepresented minorities, worked out of necessity. However, these numbers are very small and should not be generalized. A majority of students from the underrepresented minority groups (51%) reported that their parents were very involved in their high school academic experience, in comparison to 36% of whites and 20% of Asian Americans. The underrepresented minorities received the least support from their high school peers for continuing in math and science. Only 19% reported receiving strong support, in comparison with 38% of whites and 41% of Asian Americans. Teachers and counselors, on the other hand, were more involved, providing strong support to 59% of white students, to 62% of underrepresented minorities, and to 69% of Asian Americans.

PRE-PREMED PROFILE

While there were similarities in the pre-college experiences of the premed students in my sample, the profile presented here describes the majority only; there were numerous exceptions. Few of these high school students, male or female, were burdened with household responsibilities or necessary part-time employment. They had discretionary time, which they occupied to some degree with a wide range of extracurricular activities. Their parents were better educated than parents of college students nationally. The premed students were interested in science, especially biology, and they did not shy away from quantitative subjects. They took extra science in high school, especially biology, when the courses were offered, liking science and doing well in it. They began the algebra sequence early, and many advanced through Calculus I while in high school. There would be even less diversity in their science achievement by the end of high school if all their schools had offered advanced coursework in the sciences. When advanced courses are not offered, even the best students in some high schools will feel underprepared for a rigorous premed curriculum in college. These are well-rounded men and women who are pursuing their goals in a supportive atmosphere; they are distinguished largely by their interest in science and by their academic performance.

The women in this sample took math and science courses, at the advanced level, and earned high grades. With such demonstrated ability in these subjects, these women were building on their strength by taking an intensive science curriculum in college. And for the smaller number of men and women who could have had a stronger foundation for premed, Betz (1994) noted that persons may inaccurately estimate their ability in some area. "Overestimators may try and fail, but underestimators may never try at all" (p. 244). Parents can encourage their daughters (and sons) in difficult subjects by emphasizing the value in completing them more than the grades earned.

PREMED BIOGRAPHIES: OUTSIDE THE CLASSROOM

Ten of the premed students were introduced in Chapter 2, with emphasis on their family backgrounds and high school academic experience. These introductions are expanded here, with information on their life outside the classroom.

Marsha was employed more than 25 hours a week during her junior and senior years of high school. The decision to work was hers, and she had the full support of her parents. Although this was a large time commitment, she had no household responsibilities and her participation in extracurricular activities did not exceed 5 hours a week throughout high school. She had some science toys as a child but seldom played with them. She described her understanding of machines and of how to fix things as *moderate*. She never discussed her math and science courses with her parents, whom she described as *moderately* involved in her high school academic experience. Support from her counselor was strong for continuing in math and science, in contrast to the lack of support received from her peers.

Michael, too, was employed—10 to 15 hours a week in a family-owned business. He also spent 5 hours a week on household responsibilities and 10 to 15 hours a week on extracurricular activities. He demonstrated a high level of commitment to one activity, devoting 5 or more hours a week throughout high school to it. As a child he often played with the science toys, especially the building toys, that his parents bought for him. These toys may have contributed to his *great deal of understanding* of machinery. His knowledge of the premed curriculum while he was in high school was accurate but incomplete, and he took science courses in his school's honors curriculum because he thought they would help him later in college. His teachers, counselors, and peers were supportive of his interest in math and science. Many of his friends took the same courses that he took and did well in these subjects.

Emily was not employed during the school year until her senior year, when she worked 25 hours a week for a few months. She devoted more than 15 hours a week to extracurricular activities and more than 5 hours a week to a single activity for 4 years. Her household responsibilities consumed less than 5 hours a week. Her parents bought building toys for her, although she seldom played with them. She described her understanding of machinery as *moderate*. Both parents were actively involved in her academic experience, participating in her selection of courses and attending programs at school. They also encouraged her interest in science and mathematics, as did her high school teachers and counselor. Peers were less supportive.

Nora was an athlete in high school, and her extracurricular activities took 15 to 25 hours per week during the seasons of the two sports in which she participated. Her household responsibilities were limited to less than 5 hours a week, and she was not employed during the school year. She had building toys as a child and played with them often, but she had little understanding of machinery and of how to fix things. Her parents were very actively involved in her academic experience, helping her to choose courses, and their interest in her math and science performance was greater than for other subjects. She described her teachers but not her counselor as *moderately* supportive. She received little support from her peers.

Ben's major extracurricular activity in high school was band, to which he devoted 10 to 15 hours per week for 4 years, an unusually high level of commitment. He still had time to study, however, since he spent less than an hour each week on household responsibilities and he was not employed. He obtained much of his information on premed requirements from college catalogs. His knowledge of the college premed curriculum had no effect on his high school course choices, however, because there were few options open to him. He played with his science toys often as a child, yet he later had little understanding of machinery and of how to fix things. His parents were *somewhat* involved in his academic experience. They expected him to do well, but they did not steer him toward or away from science. His teachers, counselors, and peers provided no support for him at all.

Lynn was employed 20 hours a week during her senior year of high school, because she had free time and wanted to save some money for college. She spent less than 5 hours per week on household duties and was able to maintain her involvement of close to 20 hours a week in extracurricular activities. She played a musical instrument, to which she devoted more than 5 hours per week throughout high school. She had building toys as a child, which she seldom played with, and described her understanding of machines as *moderate*. Her parents did not discuss courses with her, nor did they steer her toward or away from science, but they were supportive in providing a home environment conducive to study. High school teachers and counselor were described as providing strong support, and peers were moderately supportive.

Charles was not employed until his senior year, when he worked 15 hours a week, to earn extra spending money. His parents did not object, so long as his employment had no negative effects on his academics. He spent 1 to 5 hours a week on chores around the house and more than 20 hours a week on extracurricular activities during his senior year, more than in other years. Student government was a major commitment that year; however, he had no ongoing involvement in any single activity of 5 hours or more per week over 4 years. He had science toys as a child, but these did not improve his understanding of machinery; he had *virtually no* such understanding. His parents did not steer him toward science, but they provided *a great deal* of encouragement for him to succeed in high school and made monetary sacrifices for him. He did not discuss his career interests with his friends, but his teachers made sure that he got into the math and science classes that he wanted.

Amy worked 10 hours a week during her junior and senior years, for spending money. She also devoted 15 to 20 hours weekly to extracurricular activities, especially church-related activity and community service. Her level of commitment was high, in an organization to which she was elected president in her senior year. As the oldest child in the family, her responsibilities at home were significant, too, consuming 10 to 15 hours per week. As a child, she had building toys and a microscope, with which she played often, contributing to her *great deal of understanding* of machines. Her plans for premed had no impact on her choice of high school courses. She did not discuss her course selections with her parents, but they were supportive of her choices, especially of her interest in science and math. Her teachers and her high school counselor provided strong support for her, letting her know when she did not perform as well as she should. Her peers, to the contrary, provided no support.

Chris was not employed while in high school. He participated in only two extracurricular activities, both sports, but was highly committed to them, devoting 10 to 15 hours to each in its season. As a child, he played often with the science toys that his parents bought for him. His father was deceased, and his mother encouraged him to succeed by setting a good example for him. His high school teachers and counselor were supportive of his interest in math and science, but his peers provided no support. What would he have done differently?—taken chemistry in grade 12 instead of grade 10.

Dan worked 5 to 10 hours in his junior year in a family business. He also spent more than 10 hours a week in extracurricular activities. As an athlete, he devoted close to 25 hours a week to his sports during playing seasons and participated for 4 years. Household responsibilities took 1 to 5 hours a week. He had building toys as a child, which he played with often, but had no science toys and *virtually no* understanding of machines. His parents were involved in his high school experience, and his mother, in particular, discussed course selections with him. They provided a great deal of encouragement for him to succeed, as did his high school teachers and counselor. His peers took the same courses that he took, and they supported one another.

THERE WAS NO pattern to dating frequency: Amy and Marsha dated at least once a week throughout high school; Chris, Michael, Emily, Charles, and Lynn dated less frequently than once a week early in high school but at least once a week in their senior year. While Dan, Ben, and Nora dated less frequently than once a week in their senior year, they were the students with high levels of commitment to sports and to band, activities that competed with dating for free time on weekends. It is becoming clear from the experiences of these ten premeds that they made different choices en route to a college premed program. While most had a high level of commitment to an extracurricular activity throughout high school, some did not. While most were employed at some time during the school year, some were not. While some parents were highly involved in the academic experience of these sons and daughters, others were not. These profiles underscore the array of different experiences that pre-premed students bring to college.

Chapter 4

THE PREMED PROGRAM

"My interest in science increased a lot [in college]. The more you learn, the more you understand and the more you want to learn. I was not a big science person in high school. Now I want all my classes to be science."

The premed experience is an ongoing series of choices. The individual students make tentative and then more binding decisions at each of a series of steps throughout the undergraduate program. The decision made at each point—consciously, where action is taken, or by default, when an action opportunity is passed by—increases or decreases commitment to this professional goal. Each test grade can bring with it affirmation or doubt of scientific aptitude in particular and overall ability in general. Affirming medicine presupposes some assumptions about what the profession entails and how its demands mesh with the abilities and interests that the individual brings to the match. To reach the goal of the MD degree, individuals must come to see themselves as doctors, and earlier on, as people who *can be* doctors. If instead a person perceives overwhelming obstacles from within (lack of ability in science or lack of discipline) or from without (structural or cultural constraints), then he or she will not expect ever to be a doctor. These perceptions, accurate or not, affect persistence in the premed program.

THE FIRST YEAR

The premeds took several required courses during their first year of college. While some of them entered college with advanced placement credit, most students took one semester of English (a requirement for medical school), one or two semesters of foreign language, one or two semesters of mathematics, and two semesters of chemistry in the first year. The students anticipating majoring in biology took that subject, too; other premeds completed their course schedule with electives. The first semester of college is a period of many adjustments in and out of the classroom. Even well-prepared students may experience difficulty with courses in the first year, while they are still making these adjustments. Consequently, it can be difficult for them to estimate their longer-term chances for academic success.

Science Courses

The favorite course for most of these premeds in the first year of college was not in math or science. While it may seem surprising that a majority of premed students would name a nonscience course as their favorite, their science courses at this point were those required for medical school. They were relatively large in size and consequently more impersonal. Because success in these courses is necessary in order to have any chance of admission to medical school, the experience is stressful. When asked why a course was their favorite, respondents were most likely to comment on the professor's characteristics or teaching style—the professor demonstrated knowledge of the subject matter, made the material easier to understand, created a less formal atmosphere in the course, or provided opportunities for interaction among students or between professor and students during class.

Most premed students, and all but one of those in this sample, complete a chemistry course in high school. Yet the differences between the subject as taught in high school and as taught in college are significant. When students were asked to describe these differences, a majority were able to do so easily. They reported more one-on-one interaction with teachers in high school, in smaller classes. In high school there was (far) less material covered, at a slower pace. In college there was less memorization (in general chemistry and in biology) and more emphasis on application, often requiring mathematical calculations. An extreme example of the contrast was provided by this student: "I could not apply *any* of what I learned in high school to courses here. [In high school] the teacher taught to the test, practically gave us the questions ahead of time." Chris put it more descriptively: "High school chemistry was like throwing a bullet, and [the college course] was like shooting a bullet."

Students who saw little difference between high school and college courses had taken an AP course or had taken 2 years of the subject while in high school. Fewer differences were identified between high school and college biology than in chemistry, perhaps because more of the premeds had taken a second year of biology before coming to college. Two differences that were mentioned were that more memorization of material was required in the high school course and that college tests required application of knowledge to new material.

While 60% of freshman premeds sometimes (41%) or always (19%) felt free to ask questions in their premed classes, the other 40% seldom or never felt free to do so. In large lecture classes, such as those in premed science courses taught at universities across the country, it is difficult for many students to ask questions. They may fear looking stupid when other students seem to understand or fear receiving direct criticism from the professor, who wants to maintain the momentum of the class. He or she may dismiss question attempts with "We have already covered that."

> I had no idea what the chemistry professor was talking about—ever—so to ask a question would mean he would have to re-explain everything.

> When the professor says, "but of course you know this," it makes you look foolish if you ask a question.

When fellow students also appeared lost or when the professor solicited questions or at least did not discourage them, students felt freer to raise their hands. One student described another deterrent to questions in science classes: "It is harder to ask questions in science classes because you cannot challenge someone on a formula."

As these courses usually did not build in any discussion component, student questions on course content and questions generated by the professor provided most of the interaction in class. There was a set amount of material to be covered in the course, usually in lecture format, presented by the instructor (information provider) to the students (information recipients). This style of delivery was not inconsistent with the content of the course examinations, with problems to be solved to reach the (one) correct answer. In a large lecture class, student questions may be entertained when they are few, because a few questions will not slow down the class too much. Yet, as Van der Meij (1988) noted, a single question also stands out and distinguishes the student from others, bringing unwanted attention, even while it probably contributes to the learning of the whole class. An exception to this portrait of a large, somewhat stressful classroom experience was noted by one student, suggesting that large does not have to mean impersonal: "The professor knew my name to call on me, the first time I spoke in class, even though I had never gone to see him in his office."

Some questions asked during the first and second interviews were concerned with approaches to studying and note-taking. Students who had more limited comprehension of the subject matter, or prepared less before class, or were more anxious, might attempt to include in their notes everything the professor said or wrote on the board (verbatim notes). This strategy, however, severely reduced students' listening time. Students who do not listen actively cannot make connections as the lecture progresses, and they learn less during class time. Peper and Mayer (1986) observed that "taking notes forces the learner to concentrate on the motor act of writing instead of more fully listening to the lecture" (p. 34). Students in their first year of premed studies were more likely to take verbatim notes in their science classes rather than writing in their own words what they understood from the lectures. Then they had to start learning the material outside of class. This method of note-taking is not necessarily effective. Reporting on research on study habits, King (1992) noted that "generally, students capture less than 40% of available lecture information in their notes (e.g., Hartley & Cameron, 1967; Howe, 1970) and college freshmen in particular note only about 11% (Hartley & Marshall, 1974)" (pp. 314, 316). Related to note-taking is the method of studying. When the students in my sample were asked whether they focused primarily on performance on exams (even when this meant memorizing course content without understanding it) or tried to understand course content, 61% said they tried to understand the material. This is not to suggest that they did not memorize material; rather it was not their dominant approach to learning.

In science and mathematics courses, students must have a good grasp of the material already covered in order to understand the new course content. Tobias (1990) studied the way science often is taught at the introductory level—in large classes with a lecture format. With the assistance of some graduate student volunteers from nonscience disciplines who were enrolled in some basic undergraduate science courses, she was able to document the frustration experienced by students. They reported that at certain points during a course, when the professor made a connection or used an example they did not understand, they would get lost. It then became difficult or impossible for them to get beyond that point until the confusion was clarified. When they attempted to ask questions which went beyond *how*, wishing to engage in dialogue with the instructor, their attempts were not well received, even by the other students in the class. While temporary incomprehension is a common experience among students in mathematics and science courses, students who do well in these subjects are those who are able to avoid or overcome the lingering frustration that can be caused by such moments of confusion. As one student said about college science classes: "If you don't understand, the class goes on anyway."

One explanation for the difficulty experienced by the nonscience students in Tobias's (1990) study was provided by a professor of physics, who said that he *assumed* that students in general physics had some "hands-on experience with how things work" (p. 19). This was a *hidden* assumption— that some learning of the subject had already occurred outside the course— that was not stated as a course prerequisite. Students who lacked that background would be highly disadvantaged, because they would not understand the examples introduced to *clarify* difficult, abstract concepts. Those who were familiar with applications of science were able to use that knowledge to their advantage. When our students were asked about their understanding of machines and how to fix things, such as cars, radios, and stereos, there was no consensus overall, but few students (11%) admitted having a great deal of such understanding.

Basic science courses taught to college freshmen and sophomores require that students learn the appropriate procedures for solving problems. Unlike some of the humanities and arts courses these students also take, creativity on an assignment is not likely to be rewarded. The exam format provides one illustration: Wilson, Gass, Dienst, Wood, and Barry (1975) noted that essay exams, uncommon in these science courses, communicate to students the professor's "belief in the open-ended, unfinished nature of knowledge" (p. 39) and suggest that there is no single correct answer. Premeds recognize that most of their science professors will grade exams against a standard, where there is a single answer and one or a very small number of accepted ways to get that answer. As one student in general physics noted: "With only three questions on the test, I was anxious about getting one wrong." Riesman (1980) noted that in the "high-consensus fields" of mathematics and the natural sciences, even the best students are more likely to accept the grade awarded by the professor and less likely to make the case that there is another way to arrive at an answer or that the professor was biased in grading the exam. Many of the premed courses lead to a subsequent course; the result is that there is a specified body of material to be covered, with little time for discussion. Frustration is experienced by students who want to understand as they go along or at least to have the pieces fit together when they reread their text or class notes.

Outside the Classroom

First-year students reported that math and science faculty were available outside of class, most likely during scheduled office hours or by appointment, but were less available than faculty in other disciplines. In their *unavailable* times, these faculty were likely to be in their laboratories. Some students who elected to major in science would later gain valuable research experience from these same faculty, finding them very available in these same laboratories where they were less accessible to first-year students. Having access to faculty, however, does not imply anything about the nature of this interaction. Contact with professors outside of class is of value to students not only in helping them improve their performance—by going over errors on recent tests or assignments, or by clarifying points made in class—but also in allowing them to discuss the subject being taught, one presumed to be of mutual interest. In the premed courses, professors may complain that too many premed students are in the course only for the grade, not for the knowledge. Professors would like students to have an intrinsic interest in their subject, rather than an approach to the subject that is largely instrumental.

Some students learn outside of class by participating in study groups. The value of study groups came to public attention after Uri Treisman (1992), a professor at the University of California, found that student success in first-year calculus was higher for those students who participated in study groups. A single student may not distinguish between the easier homework problems and those that are more complex, requiring a greater investment of time. When students meet together to work on problem sets, the group is less likely to spend excessive time on the easier problems, because someone is likely to remember that this type of problem has a quick solution. About half of this premed population were members of study groups for one or more premed courses during their first year. In these groups, a small number of students got together a few times during the semester to work on problems or to quiz one another on what they regarded as likely exam material. Some of the groups were sufficiently well organized to invite assistance from outside the group: "We would invite a chemistry professor or an upperclass student to the study group to go over problems and material we did not know." Some students who did not belong to such groups would have preferred to do so but did not know how to find a group or start one. Others felt unprepared to participate: "You have to be prepared on your own first. I'm not organized enough yet to study first, then meet."

Study time for all courses averaged 20 hours per week during the first year, but the average is misleading. At one extreme, a student reported studying only 4 hours a week, while at the other extreme, someone studied 65 hours. Michaels and Miethe (1989) noted that the relationship between the quantity of study time and grades earned is not straightforward. One would expect upperclass students to have become more effective in their use of study time and hence to be able to put in less time for the same outcome. A majority of the students spent at least 40% of their study time on chemistry, a course in which all were enrolled at that time, but only 24% of the sample did *all* of the chemistry problems. When asked to compare their performance in the course with that of other students in the class, three-quarters of all premeds interviewed rated their own performance as average or somewhat better than average.

Half the freshmen were employed part-time during the school year, working in food services or as cashiers, lifeguards, tutors, baby-sitters, sales clerks, secretaries, lab assistants, dance or tennis instructors, janitors, delivery drivers, veterinary assistants, ambulance service workers, parking lot attendants, alarm installers, and computer operators, among many other occupations. They spent 5 or fewer hours per week in extracurricular activities, on average. While time was often in short supply, limiting the extent to which they could participate in extracurricular activities, first-year premeds were likely to have performed some community service during the year.

Summing Up

These first-year premeds were asked the open-ended question: "What have been the most difficult aspects of the premed program for you?" Their responses focused on the academic program—the difficulty of chemistry; the large size of science classes; the time commitment required to succeed in this demanding curriculum; and the competition with other students. Examples of student responses included "maybe my best won't be good enough," "I'm putting forth extra effort that other students don't seem to have to," "having to plan ahead so much," and "too little time."

Not feeling comfortable in their courses and not having formed relationships with professors in these large premed classes, first-year students sometimes felt powerless in a situation where they had a great deal at stake. A majority of those interviewed were likely to have questioned their career goals and to have thought about pursuing a career other than medicine. The small number of men and women who had already left the premed program by the time of the first (and as a result, the last) interview did so because of poor performance, too much competition, dislike of chemistry, or intense time commitment coupled with a lack of interest in required courses.

> I didn't think I wanted it badly enough for the effort required.

> Medicine is too demanding; malpractice insurance is high, doctors' salaries are decreasing, and the risk from infectious disease is too great.

> I like how my parents live [both of whom are in medicine], but I don't enjoy the [premed] classes enough for the effort required.

> I am no longer heading for medical school. Practically, I can't get in and I have realized that I don't want the life of a medical student and a doctor, with the amount of time involved. I want a 9-to-5 job where I can feel good about myself.

Other students described what they saw as a stigma in leaving premed: "Would others think less of me if I quit?"

After two semesters, the average grade of all premeds in the study in the two courses that a majority completed, Chemistry I and II, was C+.

Their mean grade-point average for all courses was 2.88 on a 4-point scale—achievement lower than that required for admission to medical school. The average grades of those who began a second year in premed were C+ in the chemistry courses and 2.94 overall. While some of them were not yet succeeding in the program at the level that would yield admission to medical school, a majority of the premeds persisted to the second year.

THE SECOND YEAR

In any study such as this one, where participation was voluntary and where data were collected over a period of years, there is a possibility that the individuals who volunteered and remained involved in the study were not representative of the population as a whole. To check this, participants and nonparticipants were compared at different points in time, using SAT/ACT scores and grade-point average as measures. Premed students in the entering classes of 1989 and 1990 who did not volunteer for the study were compared at the start with the participants on their verbal and math standardized test scores. There were no significant differences between the two groups. At the close of the first year of college, premed students who had agreed to participate in the study were compared with those who had not. There was no significant difference in GPA between the two groups. Once students were enrolled in premed classes, attrition from my study came from two sources: those students who were no longer premed and whom I no longer followed, and those who did not schedule an interview, some of whom were still premed. As noted earlier, comparisons between the study participants and the premed program leavers showed a difference in college GPA, in favor of participants. This is neither surprising nor disturbing, since some students left premed, and hence this study, because they recognized that their grades were not competitive for medical school admission.

During the second year of the premed program, 96 students who were still enrolled in a premed course were interviewed. By the end of the second year, a science course was the favorite course of the majority. The premeds found it somewhat easier to ask questions in class than in the previous year, yet 32% seldom or never felt free to ask questions. A science course also was voted the most difficult course in college to date by an overwhelming majority, with courses selected as favorite or most difficult primarily because of course content. Nearly 60% reported that their interest in science had increased during the past year, 18% reported a decrease, and the rest experienced no change. Those who reported an increase often attributed it to having taken more specialized courses that tackled subject matter in greater depth or to successful performance in science courses they had completed.

The major academic event for most of these premeds during the second year of college was the two-semester organic chemistry course. They also took another science course each semester, a biology or a physics course. In the first year many of the premeds had been apprehensive about organic chemistry, and few had expected to like it. It won hands down as the most difficult course. References to the course include: "It's things you've never seen in your life" and "The volume of material was irrelevant to life as I know it" (Michael). Premeds devoted an average of 9 hours a week out of class to studying and preparing assignments for this course. Yet, in spite of its reputation as a killer course, organic chemistry was far from a disastrous experience for most of these men and women. When subjectively evaluating their performance in comparison with other students in the class, more said they did better than said they did worse. Some actually enjoyed the course and the challenge:

> Organic Chemistry II was easy for me; everything clicked.

> I understood what I read....I understood more than in general chemistry, because there is no math involved.

> Organic II was my second favorite course [of all taken thus far in college].

> My organic chemistry professor stimulated my interest [in science].

> I had feared [organic chemistry], but once I was in it, I enjoyed the challenge. I worked hard and I did well.

At least one professor supplemented the work of the class, as described by this student:

> I went to study sessions the professor held on Friday or Saturday nights from 7 to 9 P.M. [in a classroom]. [We] would ask questions, and the professor would have you work the problem on the board.

That this professor and these students gave up time on weekend evenings to participate in organic chemistry help sessions speaks highly of the professor's dedication and the students' motivation. This study group also illustrated what some students meant when they said that the premed program left them with little or no free time. While a number of students had complained about another professor teaching this course, one student said: "I loved the way he taught, and I loved the book [text]. The course wasn't difficult, and I understood it as I went along."

Yet organic chemistry *was* difficult for most students. That fact, combined with the importance of doing well, resulted in frustration with the practice of grading on the curve. In many premed science courses across universities, professors impose a grade distribution on raw test scores to approximate a bell-shaped curve. There are more grades in the middle of this distribution, C grades, than there are at either end. Several students volunteered that the average numerical score on an exam in organic chemistry was: 60, 38, 23, and even 15 (of a theoretically possible 100). This reported variation in exam averages is particularly interesting, since some of the discrepant responses came from students in the *same section* of the course. One was from a student who took the course at another university, demonstrating that low scores are not confined to a particular institution. The class average would convert to a letter grade at or near the C range.

Students learn in their required premed courses that while they want to understand everything as they go along, the volume of new and difficult material means that there will be times when they have to memorize information they do not (yet) understand. "In organic chemistry, you should memorize first and learn later." Yet there is no more time *later*, because there will always be new material to study or memorize. Furthermore, some students in the class are not so overwhelmed:

> Even though it [organic chemistry] was extremely hard, I found it very challenging and stimulating. Quite frankly, if the pressure was not an existing factor, I would have found it [to be] very much like a puzzle-type of game.

> In organic chemistry I understood what I read.

> I kept up with the reading, and I understood everything as we went along. I memorize easily and that's all it is.

Nor does the challenge of mastering (or at least memorizing) a large quantity of material end in college. Plantz, Lorenzo, and Cole (1993), referring to medical school courses, said that because of the volume of material to be covered, "those students with the sharpest memorization and retainment skills quickly rise to the top of any medical school class. . . . It is possible, however, to do well simply by studying a great deal, that is, 6 to 10 hours a day, 7 days a week" (p. 137). From a study conducted within a single medical school: "Students rank the ability to memorize as by far the most important ability needed to adjust to the work of medical school" (Bloom, 1973, p. 4). Faculty at that same institution agreed that the ability to memorize was more important for medical students than the "ability to cope with theoretical material" (Bloom, 1973, p. 78). Yet the premed students resisted memorizing.

Most students still took verbatim class notes in their second year. While a slight majority still attempted to understand the material rather than memorize it, a third of the group reported they did both, a response no doubt to the increased volume of material they were accountable for. Those who learned that they could not understand everything as they went along and would have to memorize some of it were developing a strategy they would use later in medical school, when the volume of material to be covered was far greater.

Effective use of study time is important for students who have a great deal of material to cover. These premeds were divided on the issue of rewriting class notes for premed courses; half did and half did not. They were even less likely to rewrite notes for their nonscience courses. Many (nearly two-thirds) listened to music or watched television while studying for nonscience courses but were unlikely to do so when studying for science courses. They were more likely to study throughout the term for any course than to cram before the exam, but they were more likely to cram in nonscience courses than in premed courses. A majority did not have set, designated study hours each week. In their second year, they studied 24 hours a week, on average, compared with 21 hours the year before.

The premeds chose majors primarily because they were interesting fields and secondarily to prepare for medical school coursework. These two reasons mirror a distinction made by Hearn and Olzak (1981), who suggested that students use two types of criteria in choosing majors, *intrinsic* and *extrinsic*: "Intrinsic criteria are founded upon goals of personal growth and expression. Extrinsic criteria relate to . . . post graduation objectives" (p. 197).

Prior to 1957 and the influence of *Sputnik*, over half of medical students had majored in a nonscience subject in college, taking only minimal science—those courses required for admission to medical school (Funkenstein, 1978). The science preparation of medical students increased significantly during the 1960s, a result, Funkenstein suggested, of the increased federal funding for science and a popular interest in science, both fueled by *Sputnik*. While his data were collected only from students from Harvard Medical School, these students reflected the best of the national applicant pool, receiving their undergraduate degrees from many different colleges and universities. By 1968, there was a move by premedical students away from college majors in the natural sciences and toward the social and behavioral sciences, reflecting changing conditions and priorities in the larger society during the Vietnam War. While premed students may select any undergraduate major, they must (also) have aptitude for mathematics and science.

Some students complained that much of what was covered in their required premed courses was not relevant to the practice of medicine, and they felt that these courses should not be required. Yet they are required, and a successful applicant to medical school must have mastered the contents of these courses. Another frequent complaint about this curriculum was that the students were tested too infrequently. With three tests per course per semester on average, they were tested far less frequently than in high school, and each test had a significant influence on the final course grade. This practice of infrequent testing is good preparation for medical school, however, where there may be only one comprehensive exam at the end of the course. While some students wanted more frequent testing to reduce the weight of any single test, others wanted to be tested on the material just covered and then move on to the new material. Yet in medical school, exams are based on material covered throughout the course and may also assume current knowledge of material covered in earlier courses. Medical practice, too, requires that knowledge be retained over a longer period of time. Some premed students already doubted their own retention abilities: "I think your brain takes in only so much new stuff before it throws out the old stuff."

The premeds earned better grades in biology courses than in chemistry: 59% of students who completed Biology I earned grades of B or better, as did 55% of those who completed Biology II. Only 31% and 35% earned these grades in Chemistry I and II, respectively, with grades in the laboratory sections of all of these courses higher, on average. In ensuing years, the distributions of grades in Physics I and II were close to those in biology and the grades in Organic Chemistry I and II closer to those in general chemistry. The students completing physics and organic chemistry represented a smaller and self-selected portion of those who began the premed program in their freshman year. The cumulative GPA at the end of year 2 averaged 2.97. This is higher than in the previous year, due to a large extent to some attrition from premed by students with lower grades. The GPA of those students who persisted in premed into the third year was higher, at 3.05, but lower than the 3.40 to 3.50 of individuals entering medical schools.

THE FINAL TWO YEARS

The last interview was conducted during the spring of the senior year, by which time most of those who hoped to begin medical school the next fall would have been invited for an interview or accepted for admission. Seventy-seven students were interviewed a third time, including eight who said they no longer were premed. A math or science course was still selected by most as the most difficult course, influenced by the number of science majors in this group, who took relatively few nonscience courses during their last year. The seniors studied 22 hours per week, on average, with a range from 3 to 65 hours.

A majority of those who began in premed completed the required premed courses, with over 70% completing two semesters of biology, two semesters of organic chemistry, and two semesters of physics. While a majority took one or more biology courses beyond those required and 57% majored in biology, only a small minority took any additional chemistry courses. A straightforward explanation for this difference is that medical schools already require twice as many chemistry as biology courses as prerequisites for admission. An alternative explanation, supported by the interview data, is that students particularly like the content of biology courses, and many regard this field as their reason for pursuing medical school. The same is less true of chemistry.

The senior year in college makes additional demands on students as they attempt to complete their academic programs, consisting primarily of higher-level coursework. There are decisions to be made about what will follow graduation. For students applying to medical schools there are added costs in time and money—for the applications and, for the successful applicant, for interviews that may be some distance away and scheduled at the convenience of the school. Nevertheless, more than two-thirds of these students also were employed in their last year, working on average 16 hours a week. A majority by now had had some employment experience in a health or science-related occupation. While a majority were involved in community service, time spent on extracurricular activities generally was limited, with most reporting 5 or fewer hours per week. There was no pattern to the data on leadership in college activities or organizations; 33% had no leadership experience in any organization, 33% had held positions of limited responsibility, and the remainder had held positions of greater authority.

Medical schools, like other academic programs, are ranked by outside evaluators, but relatively few applicants to medical school have the luxury of taking rank into consideration in deciding which school to attend. Indeed, many applicants are pleased to receive a single acceptance. Nevertheless, we asked the premeds to select the lowest rank of school they would attend: top 10, top 25, top 50, or *any medical school*. Responses to this question measured awareness of the level of competition in admission as well as their level of commitment to medicine as a career. Thirty-nine percent of first-year students said they were interested in attending medical school only if they could attend a school ranked in the top 50; a third of this group was interested only in top 25 schools! These men and women may not have realized that the national ranking of a medical school is only one, and not necessarily a major, factor in choosing a school. Since state medical schools give preference to residents and some state schools will not even consider any applicant from out-of-state, applicants to medical school are advised to apply (also) to their state school(s) without consideration of rank.

Among those still interested in medicine in the sophomore year, only 30% were concerned about the school's national ranking, including 12 premeds who said they would not go to medical school unless they were accepted to one of the top 25 schools. More than half of those interviewed felt more committed to medicine now than in the previous year; for most of the rest, commitment level had not changed.

Two-thirds of those interviewed a third time had questioned their career goal of medicine since entering college. A third of those interviewed had already been accepted to one or more medical schools by the time of this interview; of those who had not been accepted but were still interested in attending medical school, only one person was still concerned about medical school rankings.

MOTIVATION FOR MEDICINE

When premeds were asked in their first year about the reasons for choosing medicine as a career, the reason given most often was an interest in helping people, followed at a distance by intellectual challenge, the opportunity to make use of special talents and abilities, high-income possibilities, and interest in research. They were asked, too, about the value placed upon three specific attractions of the medical profession: the chance to live a financially secure and prosperous life, which 50% in the first year thought important or very important; the chance to gain respect from others, which was important or very important to 60%; and the chance to do good for others, which was *very* important to 83%. When asked about their interest in a medical specialty, most (92%) premeds in their first year of college had made a tentative selection. Specialties chosen most often were surgery (23%) and pediatrics (15%).

In a study of students enrolled in two medical schools, Kutner and Brogan (1980) noted that "desire to help others . . . and . . . desire for independence in your work . . . were somewhat or very important reasons for entering medicine, given by a large majority of both women and men" (p. 348). Data collected on 55,000 MCAT examinees in 1992 showed that the three reasons given most often for choosing a medical career were challenge, the opportunity to make a difference, and the opportunity to serve community needs—responses very similar to those given by the premed students in this study. In excess of 90% of women, men, whites, members of underrepresented minority groups, and members of other minority groups—in short, every category of premed student nationally—gave these three responses most often (AAMC, 1994a). The altruism motive has long been frequently cited by both men and women when asked why they selected medicine.

Those individuals who are motivated strongly by income or social recognition are less likely to find alternatives to medicine and may pursue their goal of medical school admission even when their academic achievements alone would suggest that admission is highly unlikely. When a student's commitment to the goal has weakened, because of course difficulty, poorer than expected grades, or lack of time for other interests, then it may not take very much of a push or a pull for the individual to leave premed. In these cases, the probability of attaining the goal, or the value of the goal, is too low to justify additional costs. In their second year, medicine was important or very important to 48% of the respondents because of its financial rewards; to 61% because of the respect that others have for doctors; and to 93% because medicine provides the opportunity to do good for others. These responses represent no change from the first year.

By the fourth year, there was (surprisingly) little change overall in the respondents' motivations to become doctors: 43% regarded financial security and prosperity as important or very important; 62% valued respect from others; and the chance to do good for others was regarded as important by all but one of the prospective doctors. I had expected that students motivated by financial gain would persist longer than premed students with different motivations, because there are few alternative occupations that offer the financial rewards of medicine. Yet the motivations of individual students, too, can change over time:

> Now I am looking at [medicine] more as a way to make money than as a service, more at what I can get out of it than at what I can give (from a student in the second year who later decided against medicine).

> In my first two years of college, I was in [pre]medicine because of money and prestige. Now I am more aware that many people are without adequate health care.

GENDER AND PREMED

With decreasing emphasis on gender appropriateness in high school classrooms and counselors' offices, more women are entering college with the academic foundation for a science curriculum. There is growing evidence, too, that women perform no less well than men in these courses. And with less emphasis on distinct gender roles within their homes, these women also have more family support for their choice of a medical career. Indeed, some women in this study reported that their motivation to pursue medicine originated with their parents.

Academic Performance

Women studied more during their first year of college than men did, 23 versus 19 hours per week; 11% of women, and 4% of men, spent 40 or more hours a week studying. Men were more likely to belong to study groups (56% versus 43%) and more likely to feel comfortable asking questions in class, with 23% of men and 16% of women *always* feeling free to ask questions. Yet women were more likely (48%) than men (43%) to say that a science course was their favorite course that year. Relatively few women (23%) or men (25%) did *all* of the chemistry problems. And it was the men who sought out the premed adviser with greater frequency. Two-thirds of men (67%) and 57% of women had taken advantage of this source of assistance. A pattern in these results is that men were less inclined to go it alone in their first year and were more likely to participate in study groups, ask questions in class, and seek advice.

Women received more encouragement in college from their parents to pursue premed. Perhaps these parents recognized that their daughters might encounter more opposition as they continued on their chosen career path and needed more encouragement. Support from college peers can mean not being pressured to go out when they had to study or complete assignments. It can also mean that roommates and hall residents in a dormitory or in an apartment kept quiet while others were trying to study. Both women and men received moderate to strong support from college peers, women (76%) more than men (65%).

Premed students in the study were asked, "Based upon your experience, do you agree with the opinion that men usually do better at math and science than women?" A minority of the women (34%) and of the men (30%) agreed with the statement, more agreeing *somewhat* than *strongly*. Women were more likely than men to select a science course as their favorite course in college. While few men or women perceived that gender played a large role in their premed academic experience, there were a few exceptions. Two male students commented:

> Organic chemistry was my most difficult course because the teacher did not teach to the tests, had no interest in how students did, and favored the girls [in the class].

> The professor [in organic chemistry] . . . had no time for male students.

However, a female student stated:

> Professors expect that men will do better [in math and science] and favor men over women in grading.

Why is success important? Perhaps the question seems too obvious to merit serious consideration. Or there may be more dimensions to success than are at first apparent. Premeds were asked: "Success in difficult endeavors is important to people for different reasons. Which of these statements best describes why success is important to you?" They were given four alternative responses:

1. Because success in these courses demonstrates that I am competent in difficult subjects and makes me feel good about myself
2. Because I enjoy the subject matter and want to know as much as I can about these subjects
3. Because the information in these courses will be useful to me in medical school
4. Other

Women (45%), but especially men (52%), chose the first response most often. The second response, chosen next by women (27%) and tied for third among the men (at 19%), refers to intrinsic reward. The third response is the instrumental one—valuing success for the way(s) in which it might be useful later on. This alternative was selected by 23% of women and 19% of men. These responses seem to indicate that when women have similar opportunities and encouragement to achieve in mathematics and science, they will tackle the increasingly difficult content of advanced courses and will evaluate their performance and enjoy their success in ways similar to men. A difference remains, however, in their ongoing attraction to medicine as their chosen profession; women more than men questioned their career goals during the first year in college, expressing reservations about the profession more than the science curriculum.

Yet the gender difference overall in persistence in the premed program favored women. And the attrition of premed men from the university exceeded that of women, too. A higher proportion of women than of men took the first semester of organic chemistry, a measure of persistence after the first year, and a higher proportion took physics, usually in the third year. The women earned somewhat better grades overall during the first two years of college, as measured by cumulative grade-point average (2.93 versus 2.81 in the first year, and 3.00 versus 2.91 in the second). In Biology I, men and women were equally likely to have earned grades of B or better;

the same was true in Biology I lab and in General Chemistry I and Organic Chemistry I (lecture component). Women outperformed men in General Chemistry I lab and in Physics I, but men outperformed women in organic chemistry lab. Women studied more for Organic Chemistry than men (11 hours per week versus 9) and ranked their performance as better than that of other students more often than men did. As women progressed and met with success in this demanding program, they were able to acknowledge their achievement, even when put in the competitive context this question required. These data show no science or math disadvantage for women.

While women in the second year thought science GPA would be the most important factor in the medical school admissions process, men thought it would be the MCAT score. This result suggests that respondents may have been projecting their desires onto the admission process, as men tend to outperform women nationally on the MCAT. By the close of their undergraduate education, two-thirds of both men and women had questioned their career goals and had thought of pursuing a career other than medicine. They had questioned their own abilities, often in spite of high grades, as they contemplated the hard work and competition still ahead, or they had reservations about what the profession of medicine had to offer them.

Comparative Motivations

In selecting medicine as a career, two attractions identified most often by both men and women were an interest in helping others and intellectual challenge. The third attraction provided a contrast between extrinsic and intrinsic rewards: Men listed the high-income possibility of medicine (extrinsic), while women listed the opportunity to make use of special talents and abilities (intrinsic). Both men and women overwhelmingly wanted to help others through the practice of medicine. The responses by one group of women medical students in the 1960s to a question about primary motivations for studying medicine presented a point of comparison with these premed students 30 years later: 34% said that altruism was their primary motive, 5% indicated "quest for admiration," and 5% named financial security (Cartwright, 1972, p. 204).

When premeds in the first year evaluated the importance of three rewards of the medical profession—financial security and prosperity, respect from others, and doing good for others—there was overwhelming agreement from both women and men on the desire to do good for others through the practice of medicine, with all women and 92% of men attributing importance to this motive. Women were less likely (56%) than men (65%) to value the social recognition that the profession of medicine provides and placed less emphasis on financial security, with 44% of women and 60% of men saying that was important to them. The absence of any large gender difference in the altruism motive was not because there is no such difference in their age peers overall. Beutel and Marini (1995), using data from a national sample of high school seniors, concluded that "females . . . are more likely than males to express concern and responsibility for the well-being of others" (p. 436). They noted, too, that similar findings have been obtained since the 1970s.

Among the respondents who had already identified a medical specialty of interest in their first year, men selected surgery most often and women chose pediatrics. Studies of specialty choice by medical students have found similar results: Women were more likely to select a primary care specialty (including pediatrics), while men were more likely to select surgery. Patient contact has been shown to be more important to women than to men in selecting a specialty (Bergquist et al., 1985).

One of few areas where differences were apparent in the senior year was in the rewards to be derived from medicine: While 64% of the men thought that financial security and prosperity were important or very important rewards, only 30% of women shared this view, a gap that had widened over the 4 years. As men came to value the economic rewards of medicine more, women valued them less. The social rewards of medicine did not differ by gender, with 61% of women and 64% of men attributing importance to those rewards. Leserman (1981), having reviewed much of the research on this subject, concluded: "In studies of medical students, medical applicants, and physicians, women have been shown to be much less interested in high income and status than men" (p. 35). And 98% of the women and all the men said that the altruistic rewards of medicine were important to them. Women were much more likely than men to have been involved in some community service activity (not necessarily health- or hospital-related) during the last year of college. Some medical schools place positive value on applicants having worked for pay or having actively volunteered (as opposed to merely observing doctors at work) in a medical department of a hospital and/or worked in a science laboratory. No gender difference was found in this sample, with just under half of men and women having had that experience.

Views on Gender, Family, and Employment

Five items used in or adapted from previous surveys of college graduates were included during the first and third interviews, monitoring changes in attitudes during the undergraduate years. Students were asked to select among five response alternatives, from *agree strongly* to *disagree strongly*, to indicate their reactions to these items:

TABLE 4.1. Attitudes on Work and Family, by Gender (Agree or Strongly Agree)

	Freshmen		*Seniors*	
Preferential treatment	15%	17%	37%	37%
Equivalent place	97%	100%	100%	96%
More day care	97%	85%	100%	89%
Employed mother	88%	56%	90%	78%
Achievements of women	83%	79%	94%	93%

1. Because of past discrimination, women should receive preferential treatment in hiring practices (preferential treatment).
2. Women should assume an equivalent place in business and all the professions along with men (equivalent place).
3. There ought to be more day-care institutions for children so that both parents can participate in paid work and public activities (more day care).
4. An employed mother can establish just as warm and secure a relationship with her children as a mother who is not employed (employed mother).
5. The achievements of women in history have not been emphasized as much as those of men (achievements of women).

This last item was included as a more general measure of orientation toward women's issues. The data in Table 4.1 combine agree and strongly agree responses to these items.

These data, even those from students completing their first year in college, show that male premeds were not unaware of some of the concerns that women face more directly. The largest gender gap was obtained in the first interview, in response to the most personal item, concerning the hypothetical relationship between a child and an employed mother. The gap narrowed considerably over the next 3 years, as men changed their views on this matter. Two other changes in the attitudes of men and women concerned the implications of past discrimination against women and the public emphasis placed on the achievements of women. That substantially more respondents of both sexes agreed with these statements in their last year of college than in their first year is likely a consequence of having discussed these or similar issues in their college coursework.

COMPARISONS BY RACE

While gender has some impact on the various aspects of the premed experience, so, too, does race. In the first year, 42% of non-Hispanic whites (whites) earned grades of B or better in General Chemistry I, compared with 78% of Asian Americans and 19% of premeds from underrepresented minority groups. The Asian American students more often had taken extra science courses and calculus in high school, contributing to a stronger foundation for chemistry. At the close of the first year, Asian Americans earned the highest grades overall, with 63% having grade-point averages of at least 3.00, in comparison with 44% of whites and 21% of underrepresented minorities. The Asian American premeds were somewhat more likely to have participated in study groups for first-year premed courses (50%), compared with 46% of whites and 38% of underrepresented minorities.

A majority of all three groups were questioning their goals and thinking of a career other than medicine: 69% of Asian Americans, 68% of whites, and 60% of underrepresented minorities. The Asian Americans were most likely (50%) to report receiving strong support from college peers for continuing in premed, in comparison with whites (37%) and underrepresented minorities (14%). As nearly all premeds wanted to help others through medicine, the remaining types of attraction to medicine that could differentiate among groups were financial and social rewards. In the first year, the financial rewards were most appealing to whites, with 56% rating those rewards as important, compared with 38% of the other two groups. Members of the underrepresented minorities were least likely (33%) to value social rewards, in contrast to 69% of Asian Americans and 66% of whites who valued these rewards.

By the close of the second year, the motivation for medicine had changed somewhat. Financial motivation had declined for whites, with 49% saying this was important or very important; declined for Asian Americans, to 21%; and increased for underrepresented minorities, to 50%. The social rewards of medicine, too, increased for underrepresented minorities; 44% now said this was an important attraction, compared with 57% of Asian Americans and 62% of whites. Over 85% of premeds in all three groups placed importance on the altruistic rewards of medicine.

Race was not a factor in *always* feeling free to ask questions in premed classes in the second year; this response was given by 17% of whites, 14% of Asian Americans, and 11% of underrepresented minorities. Nor did race play a large role in leading premeds to question their career goals: 68% of whites had questioned medicine as their goal, compared with 64% of Asian Americans and 61% of underrepresented minorities. Perhaps the largest difference across groups in the second year was in academic performance.

At the close of the second year, 63% of Asian Americans had cumulative grade-point averages of 3.00 or higher, compared with 48% of whites and 19% of underrepresented minorities.

SOCIAL ASPECTS OF PREMED

The social aspects of premed include support and discouragement received from others, as well as comparison and competition with peers.

Social Support

While some students remained in premed only or primarily because of parental support for the goal, this was more common early in college than during the later years. While parents' support for continuing in premed was usually characterized as moderate or great, nine students said they would leave premed if they did not have parental support. Support from others in this process is not always beneficial in the long run, however. Support from peers and family can validate a student's efforts, sending the message that someone else thinks I can do this, but also can keep the less qualified student identified longer as premed. The student who is above average, even slightly so, can benefit from such support if the result will be the increased effort which comes from renewed confidence.

Once in college, the premeds had access to a premedical adviser and were encouraged to meet with her early to review requirements. While a majority of students reported favorable contact with the adviser, those whose experience was less favorable tended to be students who were not doing well. Some were unreceptive to suggestions that they have a backup plan in case they were not admitted to medical school. Even in the later stages of occupational choice, a few of these college students still had not learned to take responsibility for their own futures. Some students did not want to hear that they might not be admitted to medical school, despite poor performance: "The premed adviser made me cry; after my first semester, when I had done poorly in general chemistry [earning a failing grade], she suggested that I pursue other careers." An extreme example was cited by one student, who said about the premed adviser: "I think it's her job to help students get into medical school even if their grades and scores are mediocre." This student, even at the end of college, had not yet appreciated how much of the admission decision is based on academic performance, especially in required courses—factors beyond the control of any adviser. One person suggested that the university hire additional staff "who know thoroughly all routes to medical school," expressing a belief that what was lacking was information—that there is a way to determine *exactly* what it takes to be admitted, and that this information was not made available to this student and to his classmates. He failed to acknowledge that in a competitive process, to which each medical school brings (slightly) different interests, there is a subjective element in the admissions process that will remain beyond prediction.

Social Comparison

Personal insight into our abilities comes through interaction with other people—directly, when a course instructor assigns a grade, or indirectly, when a student begins to notice that some others in the study group know how to tackle certain math or science problems while she or he does not. For some students, this inability to solve the problems persists week after week, signaling a weakness in this required subject, a subject in which the final grade matters a great deal. If a premed student cannot improve performance with added effort, he or she will alter personal aspirations or be miserable, living daily with the knowledge of not having the necessary ability to reach the goal. Getting into medical school and eventually practicing medicine are valued goals not only to those in premed but in the larger society as well, since the medical profession continues to be regarded as the most prestigious occupation. This level of social recognition by itself puts pressure on some premed students, who feel that changing career paths, even though a personal decision, will let down the larger society. What they probably mean is that they will let down their parents and those other family members who hope to see them become doctors.

A visible manifestation of social comparison is found in course grades. "Students want not only to discover how well they did on the exam, but also to find out that they did well" (Gruder, 1977, p. 23). They are making social comparisons in the hope of maintaining or increasing self-esteem. Two approaches to test grading are criterion referencing and norm referencing. A criterion-referenced test compares each student's performance against an absolute standard; receiving an A grade requires that the student answer 90% or more of the questions correctly. The test is constructed so that a student in the class who has fully mastered some finite amount of material, such as that covered in a course, *could* answer all of the questions correctly. A norm-referenced test, in contrast, compares the performance of a particular student against performances of all other students in the class. The best are awarded A grades, somewhat weaker performances receive Bs, and so on, down through the grading scale.

With norm referencing, the student with the best exam may answer far fewer than 90% of the exam questions correctly, if other students knew even less. If the same test were given to more advanced students, the numerical scores would be higher, but the grade distribution, when translated to letter grades, might not differ by very much. A college freshman who entered an introductory class with the advantage of a strong background in the subject, or engaged a very good tutor, or gave up all other interests to study this subject, could earn a higher numerical score on a 100-point scale than beginning students usually earn. He or she, in effect, would raise the numerical score required to earn an A on the test. As noted earlier, many science and mathematics courses use norm referencing, referred to as *grading on the curve*. The instructor attempts to fit the grade distribution of the class to a *normal*, bell-shaped curve. The student just described would *break the curve* with an unusually high numerical score. With norm referencing, grades become a more ambiguous indicator of performance until the students have some basis for comparison, which they get when the professor provides information on the distribution of grades for the whole class. Not all students perceive their score as equivalent to the letter grade assigned, however: "I got a B, but it is really a D". Michael said that he had a numerical average in Organic Chemistry II of 70; the professor wanted to give him an A+ for this superior performance but the university grading scale stopped at A, so Michael received an A in the course.

Norm referencing tends to increase the already high level of competition among premed students and contributes to the fear that fellow students in the first science courses in college will earn their As primarily because of their superior high school background in this subject. And students have less incentive to help one another. A student who is at or near the top of the class still may be willing to help a weak student, because the strong student is not likely to jeopardize class standing in doing so. Other students, expecting B− or B grades at best, will be more uncertain about what level of performance on a test is *good enough* to sustain or improve their course grade. If the student who is helped outperforms the helper, the latter student may fall from the more highly valued B range to the less valued C range. One student expressed his dissatisfaction with norm-referenced grading:

> In high school, more emphasis was placed upon understanding concepts. Here it is how well you understand in comparison to others in the course. Professors will not give you tests that you can finish—they admit that. Information can be applied in different ways, and you do not know ahead of time which of these ways will earn you a higher grade.

The assignment of grades in a course does not have to encourage competition among students, as it does in these science courses. It does not do so in most pre-college classrooms or in college classes where the number of possible As is not fixed. While it may appear that such norm-referenced grading would be used more often in humanities courses, where a single correct answer is not the measure of effectiveness, these courses rarely use a curve.

The theory of social comparison processes (Festinger, 1954) posits that when objective measures of ability are unavailable, individuals will use more subjective measures to make comparisons with the abilities of others who are like them in some relevant way. We want to choose reference groups that make us feel successful after comparing ourselves favorably to others. Our self-esteem is enhanced if these others are high performers. This poses a problem for many premed students in a selective academic environment, since there will be a shortage of others with whom they can make favorable comparisons. Those at the midpoint of the grade distribution can compare themselves favorably with those closer to the bottom, but they do so with the knowledge that those close to the bottom will most definitely not be accepted by a medical school, and hence such comparisons are not very meaningful. There are circumstances under which individuals choose reference groups whose members differ from them in significant ways: "One such situation occurs when the attraction of the group is so strong, for other reasons, that the member continues to wish to remain in the group" (Festinger, p. 137). This situation describes the circumstance of many premed students.

Comparison with fellow students extends beyond an individual test or course; students also are ranked within their cohort. A frequent request made of a college dean's or registrar's office is for information on class rank. That such comparisons are made across an entire cohort of students who have completed a certain number of semesters in the institution, regardless of the content and difficulty of courses taken, might appear to diminish their usefulness. Nevertheless, the tendency to compare oneself with others who are in some way similar is evident, even when the medical school, graduate school, or potential employer does not request rank information.

By the end of the second year of college, most premed students have finished six of the eight required semester-long science courses and are more than halfway through college. In the junior year, most completed the final premed requirements and took the MCAT. They also seriously researched medical schools to which they planned to apply. The reference groups for advanced premeds consist of their competitors for places in medical school in the year when they will apply. They cannot put faces on these competitors, so this reference group exists only in the aggregate, *out there*. This group becomes salient when the student is taking the MCAT or completing medical school applications. Premeds compete for acceptance to graduate and professional programs with students from colleges nation- and worldwide, with insufficient information about these other students and colleges for them to constitute a meaningful reference group. Those not at the top of their graduating class hope that their grades in the required courses will carry more weight with admissions committees than those of applicants from less competitive institutions, hoping that a B grade would be equivalent to an A at many other schools or a C to a B at those schools. Their question, which had no simple answer at that stage, was: "How good is good enough?" In the final year of college, premeds think, too, about what they want from medicine and determine how much they value the rewards they expect to receive from practicing medicine.

The Competition

Competition is a fact of life when only one in three applicants will gain admission to medical school. Yet students in the same premed program had different views on the competition:

> Engineering students are breaking the curve [in general chemistry] and should not be in this class.

> It's really competitive, and I am not an overly competitive person.

> The level of competition is very high among premed students; they do not share notes, for example.

> I don't feel that it was the material [in premed courses] that was so hard. Instead, I found the fact that these were such important classes with a lot of competition was what made it difficult.

> It's a competitive environment but not excessively so. No one is blowing up labs or stealing books from the library, like at some other places.

Others were motivated by the competition: "Biology [taken in the first year] was my favorite course. I got the highest grades." When asked about the positive aspects of the premed experience, one premed responded: "Doing well in courses that others are scared of. I, too, was scared of these courses when I started." While one student said he would prefer *cooperative learning*, other students claimed to have found it, at least outside the classroom:

> I liked the unity among premed students.

> There was a close bond with other students while taking the MCAT and preparing for it.

> Premed students ahead of you can tell you what to do that works..., advise you.

Premed students stick together and help each other.

Camaraderie with other premed students—that's been really neat.

A very small number of students did not experience much competition *or* cooperation, largely because they consistently performed very well and did not need to rely on others to understand course material. One student, after he had been accepted to medical schools, commented:

I'm thankful that things worked out well, although I didn't doubt they would. If all students here who want to could get into medical school, that would be OK with me. I don't see myself competing with them.

Succeeding when the level of competition is intense may instill in the successful person a sense of superiority that is not so compatible with the rapport that patients value from their doctor. One student said that she found medical students to be arrogant, going on to say that some medical school faculty she had met viewed this arrogance as a by-product of acceptance to medical school. The process is such that not only did the better students advance to the next step but along the way some individuals who started out only wanting to become doctors came to value the competitive process, because they emerged from it victorious.

Those science professors who wish to provide a more interactive and less competitive climate for student learning may find that decisions about class size, content, and structure are not theirs to make. Texts may be selected by a committee, and class size is dependent on faculty availability and student demand. The introductory courses can be structured as "pumps" or as "filters" (Steen, 1987, p. 19), pumping students into the science pipeline or screening them out. If the class size is large, it is very difficult for a professor to provide the level of attention and assistance to some students that may be required for the pump to work.

MEDICINE AND SCIENCE

Students of science learn methodologies, ways of thinking about the phenomena they are investigating, and ways of designing research so that their teachers now and their colleagues later on will accept their findings. Medicine, while science-based, is also an art, as it is practiced by specific doctors interacting with specific patients. Science does not dictate what to do in treating each patient; those decisions are the result of the professional judgment of the doctor. So, when premed students complained that much of what they were studying in their required courses was not relevant to medicine, they were saying more than they realized. While they were speaking about the lack of direct application of the content of chemistry and physics courses and the uselessness later of the formulas they were trying to memorize, there is also a seam between the scientific and the clinical aspects of medicine. Students who were more interested in the clinical aspects than in some combination of research and practice were more mindful of the distinction. Research science as a career differs from medicine in its social context, too. Research scientists work in an environment peopled primarily by other scientists and support personnel. Medical doctors, on the other hand, interact primarily with patients, delivering a valued service directly to them. Indeed, this contact with people is what motivates many young men and women to become doctors. Consequently, premed students who focus primarily on the clinical aspects of medicine will perceive an additional gap between their science courses and their professional goals that premed students with a research interest will not see.

PREMED BIOGRAPHIES: THE COLLEGE YEARS

While these ten premeds took most of the same courses, their academic and out-of-class lives were different. They all did well in science, but some had intellectual interests that competed with science for their attention. These students varied, too, in their perceptions of the difficulty of the premed program.

The First Year of College

Marsha did not find general chemistry difficult, having covered most of this material in her single chemistry course in high school. She attempted all the chemistry problems but did not belong to any study groups. Describing the difference between biology courses in high school and in college, Marsha said that in high school the teacher would go over a process but would not get into the chemistry behind the process, as her professor did in college. She studied 30 hours a week during her first year, was employed, and earned a GPA greater than 3.50. She was in the minority in not questioning her career goals during the first year and one of only five who, when asked to describe the most difficult aspects of the premed program, said there were *none*. She liked science a great deal and would take only science courses if she could. "I would rather read science than a novel." She was attracted to medicine primarily by the financial rewards and the opportunity to do good.

Michael participated in study groups for one or more premed courses and earned As in both semesters of general chemistry, his favorite course that year, and also in general biology. His GPA exceeded 3.50. Yet even he did not always feel free to ask questions in class. He was in the minority in not taking verbatim notes, trying instead to take notes in his own words. He described his high school chemistry course as only average, qualitative rather than quantitative. Perhaps that is why he attempted all the chemistry problems in his first college course. He studied 15 hours a week and was employed. Michael valued his success in the first year because he was succeeding in this difficult program. He had questioned his career goals: "Other people are having fun and I am not." The social and altruistic rewards were very important to him.

Although *Emily* described her high school background in chemistry as very good and she spent most of her 15 study hours a week in the first year on general chemistry, she did not do as well as she had expected in the lecture portion of that course, earning a C– in the first semester. She did only those problems that were assigned, but she was conscientious in her work: "You must understand each step [of the problem] perfectly. . . . You must work a problem to get the answer in order to go on to the next step of the problem." She participated in study groups with other students in her residence hall. Comparing high school and college chemistry, she said: "It moves a lot faster here; a whole year of high school chemistry was covered here in 2 weeks. You must understand the material perfectly." Her GPA in the first year was a B–. The financial, social, and altruistic rewards of medicine were all very important to her in the first year, but the difficulty with chemistry led her to question a medical career.

Nora began her first semester taking general chemistry and honors biology, although her favorite course that year was in history, because "it made us think." Much of chemistry was a review for her, as she had taken 2 years of the subject while in high school, yet she still did all the chemistry problems. She completed her first semester with a B+ in general chemistry and a B+ grade-point average overall. She participated in study groups only once or twice, preferring to study alone: "I need to cover what *I* am unsure about." She seldom felt free to ask questions in class: "When the pace slows down I can ask questions, but it seldom slows down." She was sure of her interest in science but uncertain about medicine as her career goal and said in the first year that her interest was in medical research.

Ben said that financial and altruistic rewards were very important to him. He studied 20 to 25 hours a week and did not participate in study groups: "I tend to get distracted with others; that can lead to me helping others, with less return to me." Although his background in chemistry was not very strong, he did most (but not all) of the chemistry problems, and he earned an A in general chemistry. "High school chemistry was fed to us slowly, introduced as something completely unknown. . . . In college, familiarity was assumed, or at least that you would comprehend quickly. Things seldom were repeated." He was able to learn the material in general chemistry while it was being taught, rather than taking verbatim notes and learning the material later. Even with his strong performance, however, he did not always feel free to ask questions in class. He valued his success because these were difficult courses. He questioned his career goals, less because he might not succeed than because he had interests beyond medicine and the choice was difficult for him to make.

Having completed 2 years of chemistry in high school, *Lynn* took honors general chemistry in college, earning B and A grades in the two semesters. Yet even in the smaller honors section, she did not always feel free to ask questions: "When the pace is too rapid, you can't get your thoughts together to ask questions." She did all the problems in chemistry, took verbatim class notes, and studied 30 hours a week, alone, so that she could set her own pace. She earned nearly a 3.50 GPA in her first year. In comparing her high school and college chemistry courses, Lynn said that her second chemistry course in high school was quantitative, like the college course, but the teacher gave weekly tests on "little bits of material" that had been covered in class. "In college, professors expect you to go beyond the lectures. It makes a difference that professors but not high school teachers are researchers." She described support from college peers as *moderate*, saying that other science students were less supportive because they were competing with her. None of the three types of rewards were very important to her. Like Ben, she questioned medicine because other career options were attractive, too.

Chris was disappointed in his grades in General Chemistry I and II, even though he did all the problems. He studied with others, informally and in study groups. The benefits of the group were to increase his understanding of the material and to increase the time he spent studying—to 35 hours a week. Yet he earned less than a 3.00 in his first year, a performance that led him to question his career goals *often*. He attributed his C grade in first-semester chemistry to having forgotten much of his high school course, taken 3 years earlier. His favorite course in the first year was a math course; he earned a good grade and he could apply what he learned. The only attraction to medicine that was very important to him was doing good for others.

In her first year, the financial, social, and altruistic rewards of medicine all were very important to *Amy*, and she enjoyed the prestige associated with premed. Unlike many of her fellow premeds, chemistry was her favorite subject because she found it "easier to understand than other classes." Yet her grades, in this subject and overall, were below average. She attributed her poor grade in chemistry to studying too little. She did some of the problems and studied only 8 hours a week for all courses. Her study strategy was memorizing to perform on exams. She described the college chemistry course as "very abstract." "Professors introduce material that you don't need to know. They are so advanced . . . they have difficulty relating to freshmen."

Charles hit his stride in premed courses only after the first semester, when he earned a C in General Chemistry I (but over 3.00 overall). He described his high school course as *fair*, requiring a great deal of memorization, with only a few labs during the year. He admitted that his attitude in General Chemistry I was negative; he did not like the professor, although his tests were fair. He did not feel comfortable asking questions in such a large class. He had peer support in college: "Most of my friends are premed, so they understand. People in other programs are supportive, too, because they think it [premed] is tough." Doing good for others was his only very important attraction to medicine; his goal was to be a general practitioner, and he had not questioned his career goals.

Dan completed general chemistry and two semesters of biology in his first year; his lowest grade across the 8 courses (lectures and labs) was B+, and his GPA was between A– and A for the year. Yet even he said he "wondered if he would make it" to medical school. He attributed his success in these courses to high motivation and hard work: "I was always solving problems." He spent 35 hours a week studying and preparing assignments. He was now rooming with another premed student, after having been assigned to a roommate with other, more social, priorities. His greatest difficulty with the premed program: "the time demands, a never-ending workload until summer." Only the altruistic reward of medicine was very important to him.

The Second Year

By her second year, *Marsha*'s interest in science had increased even more. She studied 20 hours a week, less than in the previous year, and now wrote fast enough to take notes verbatim and *then* add her own comments. She was interested in organic chemistry and "never missed a class." Although she kept up with the material, she said the course was made more difficult because "the professor did not plan on our doing well and would include only 30% of familiar material on exams." The financial and social rewards of medicine had declined in importance, but the opportunity to do good for others remained a strong attraction to medicine. Success in the premed program was important to her because she enjoyed the subject matter and wanted to learn as much as she could about these subjects. She earned B+ through A grades in organic chemistry and biology, with an A– GPA overall.

Michael's performance during the second year was very strong. He earned A– and A grades in organic chemistry and As in biology. Yet he did not necessarily enjoy all the premed courses: "No one getting out of organic chemistry feels it has been a good experience." He was one of few premeds to keep a study schedule, where certain hours were devoted to studying science courses. He studied 20 to 25 hours a week and was employed. "Now I [may] study 8 or 9 hours in a row, and study with someone for my science courses." The rigor of the program frustrated him during the second year: "How can I go through this for 6 more years? I have more respect for doctors now because of how much they have to know, yet I know some doctors and I wonder how they got through."

When asked during the first interview whether she expected to like her remaining premed courses, *Emily* said that she expected to dislike organic chemistry very much: "I've heard how hard it will be; it's a weed-out class." Yet the next year she earned an A in the first semester of the course and identified it as her favorite course taken that year. "It's like a puzzle, not memorization like general chemistry but more like art than science. I enjoyed the final exam. . . . I studied 4 to 5 hours per day, seven days a week, for organic chemistry," and she reported studying a total of between 45 and 50 hours each week in her second year. She also earned an A– in biology. Her approach to studying for her science courses was completely different from her study habits in other courses. For sciences she rewrote her class notes, studied without TV or music, throughout the semester, on a study schedule, and did not cram before tests. Financial security, social recognition, and doing good for others still were very important attractions to medicine in her second year. Her interest in science had increased, because she was doing better, and her commitment to medicine had also increased, although she still questioned her career goals. She said she was getting more scared, because she wanted to be a doctor but was concerned that with "so many more people trying to get in," there would not be a place for her.

After a summer course that allowed her to observe practicing physicians, *Nora* became *sure* of medicine. Yet she did not do well in Organic Chemistry II. She said about organic chemistry, her only premed course that year: "There was *so* much information; you can't always tell what is important." She was able to maintain an overall GPA of nearly B+, in spite of that course.

By the second year, all three types of reward had become less important to *Ben*. His interest in science had increased, and both his favorite and his most difficult course were in the sciences. He studied only 10 to 12 hours a week and earned an A– GPA for the year. His study habits were the same in science as in other courses—he did not rewrite notes, sometimes listened to music or TV, crammed before tests, and had no study schedule. He still questioned his career goals, but medical school rank no longer was important.

Lynn said that organic chemistry (honors section) was her most difficult course in the second year, "the first real college course I took. . . . The professor was really brilliant." She earned a B, while studying 25 hours a week for this course, 50 hours total for all courses. She took both organic chemistry and physics in the second year. Her interest in science had decreased, and she selected a nonscience major that had been rewarding because it provided her with (more) opportunity to interact with faculty. "I don't like the atmosphere of science classes. The professors make you feel stupid; the average grade is so low." After a summer internship working with physicians, she became more interested in medicine. She questioned her career goals less often at this time, but when she did, it was not from feelings of personal inadequacy. She recognized that other premeds were going through the same thing and wondered whether it was worth it. Her cumulative grade-point average was B+.

By the end of his second year, *Chris* was having doubts about his ability to handle medical school, because of his performance in college to date. His specific concern was with his general chemistry grades, as his other science grades—in biology and in physics—were As and Bs. Unlike most of his peers, he did not take organic chemistry until his junior year. He was getting discouraging advice from medical students and from doctors, who told him not to go into medicine because he "would not have enough time for a life." His response: "I'm not listening." He had begun working in a hospital, as an orderly, and he studied 30 hours a week. He rewrote his notes after class, studied throughout the term, and had a designated study schedule. Medical school rank was unimportant to him, and he expected cumulative GPA to be the factor weighted most heavily during the admissions process. He now had a B average overall. The financial rewards of medicine had become important by this time.

By the second year, the prestige and altruistic attractions of medicine had lessened somewhat in importance for *Amy*, but the financial rewards were still very important. Her interest in science had decreased, and she found it "not as much fun" as she had previously. Like Chris, she did not take organic chemistry that year but took Physics I and II. She changed her study habits, studying in the library instead of in her room, and she worked on one subject at a time, in greater depth. By that time she was experiencing doubts about being admitted to medical school, because of her college grades thus far.

Charles said that in Organic Chemistry I, the lectures were given "at breakneck speed. The professor started slow and took off. The lab is frustrating; some students give up. I didn't give up; I could work for 4 hours and still get nothing." Charles reported that the second semester of organic chemistry was even worse, the most difficult course so far. He earned a C+ grade. "The professor was a lot harder [than in the first semester] and the content was so abstract. There is a mystique about premeds and organic chemistry; it's supposed to make or break you. Before exams I'd get the jitters and would eat packets of Tums during exams." In his second year, his favorite course was in his major, in the social sciences. He had thought of giving up on medicine, because he was not doing as well as he would like and did not like "not knowing where you stand in a course." He doubled his study time between the first and second year—from 20 hours a week to 40. His cumulative GPA at the end of the year was 3.33. The only reward that was important to him was doing good for others. "I used to see medicine as glamorous; now I see it as really tough."

Dan's favorite course that year was not in science, although he said that his interest in science had "increased dramatically." "My knowledge [of science] is growing and I am learning more ways to apply science to medicine. I'm learning how the pieces fit together. We are learning these things [referring to the content of required courses] for a reason." He worked for a doctor during the summer and now had "a more realistic view of medicine." Doing good for others was still the most important of the three attractions to medicine. Organic Chemistry I was his most difficult course that year, because "the professor was not well-organized." Yet he still earned B+ and A grades in that course, and still had between an A– and A GPA overall.

IT IS APPARENT that the academic experience of the ten premeds was influenced by their background in chemistry and by their performance in the required premed chemistry courses. A better-than expected grade can increase a student's overall interest in science. Alternatively, the difficulty and volume of a course's content can cause a premed to reconsider her or his choice of profession. It is also apparent that the selection of strategies for succeeding in premed—study groups, doing more problems, note-taking—is idiosyncratic, with no single set of behaviors being right for everyone.

Chapter 5

PERSISTING AND REACHING THE GOAL

"After seeing an emergency room first-hand, I can't imagine doing anything else."

Some of the men and women who started in premed finished college relatively satisfied even without gaining admission to a medical school. They had found a preferred alternative to medicine. It was not low science grades that prompted them to search for other options. They were excited by coursework in another field or desired to devote less of their life to a career than medicine would require. What about the others? Some students selected medicine as their goal but lacked the aptitude for science. If they changed directions quickly enough and moved into a curriculum in which they could be more successful, premed was not such a bad experience. Those who persisted in premed and elected to major in a science without having a strong aptitude for it fared the worst. Their overall grade-point averages were depressed because of their major. Because these individuals did not change direction soon enough or did not realize what level of performance would be required to be an attractive applicant to medical school, their college record did not present an attractive credential for other opportunities. While some students shifted their occupational goals from medicine to law, public health, research, or business, others had more limited options upon completing college.

Between those who were admitted to a medical school (or found an equally attractive alternative) and those who invested too much in an unrealizable goal were those students whose future direction was still undecided upon graduation from college. Some would reapply to medical school the next year, and some again the year after that. Others would move on to new goals. For these individuals the highly competitive selection process, which leaves able, altruistic, motivated men and women unable to move to the next step in their career progression, exacted a high price.

Premeds can obtain information on their chances of being accepted to medical school by comparing their present performance with those of premeds admitted in the previous year. Information about recent admits provides current premed students with positive or negative reinforcement of their choice of profession. Most of our premeds during their last interview cited their nearness to the goal of medical school, rather than successes to date or growing interest in science, as the factor most responsible for increasing their interest in a career in medicine. As Bandura (1977) noted, persons who expect to be effective in reaching a particular goal will put forth greater effort over a longer time and will be willing to address adversity more than others whose "efficacy expectations" are lower (p. 80). It may be the case, however, that these expectations are based on inaccurate perceptions. Individuals who expected to succeed because they *tried so hard* were neglecting the more objective data on the intermediate achievements required to reach the long-term goal. The rare and fortunate student near the top of the scale on multiple ranking dimensions (especially grades and MCAT) is in a position to rank schools to which she or he has been accepted, attempting to maximize desired characteristics in a school.

PERSISTING TO THE SECOND YEAR

The ongoing process of pursuing medicine as a professional goal, as it has been portrayed in the tentative stage of career exploration, is not so much an evaluation of medicine against various options at each stage of the process as a comparison between continuing and not continuing in premed. At the close of the first year of college, primary factors influencing the choice are grades in the required premed courses to date, the degree to which the individual's view of herself or himself in the future is connected to medicine (measured by how early the initial choice was made), and the attractiveness of some other alternative. There are few other reasons not to continue at this point. Students who find courses difficult but are getting good grades have the satisfaction of doing well in difficult subjects. They can keep alive the possibility of medical school at no cost.

Students who enrolled in another premed course in their second year of college were classified as persisters at time 1. There were 126 persisters; 18 students chose other goals. The remainder had left the institution and could no longer be followed; their data are not included here. While the number of nonpersisters at time 1 was small, and some of them did not complete an interview, it is all the more noteworthy that some of the differences between the two groups are so pronounced.

In the following analyses, comparisons between the two groups, which are described as "more" or "less" likely or which exhibit more or less of a certain characteristic, should not be interpreted as statistically significant. The smaller number of nonpersisters for whom we have interview data, and the restricted variation in some of these variables, may not yield statistically significant results, even when there is a noticeable difference. Comparisons that report differences using quantitative data, however, such as those on GPA, course grades, and SAT scores, do reflect the results of significance tests, although the tests are used only to show the relative magnitude of these differences. Since I am not generalizing from a sample to a population, such tests are not really appropriate.

Differences in Pre-College Experiences

There were no differences in family structure (one- or two-parent), family size, or birth order between those who remained in premed after the first year and those who did not. One interesting finding was that all of the *only* children persisted to the second year. There were no differences in the educational attainment of mothers or fathers, but students whose mother or father was a physician were more likely to be found among the persisters. There were no gender differences at this point but some differences across racial and ethnic groups: all of the African American and Asian American students and the single Native American student persisted, while there was attrition in the Hispanic and non-Hispanic white groups. The numbers in some of these groups, however, are very small.

A majority of persisters and nonpersisters (66% to 67%) attended public high schools. Experiences in high school that increased the likelihood of persistence included having taken physics, honors-level chemistry, or one or more advanced science courses. Of the 23 students in the total sample who took a second year of chemistry while in high school and the 6 who took a second physics course, *all* persisted in premed beyond the first year. In contrast, completing a second biology course did not distinguish between the two groups. Advanced-level (honors, AP, or college) courses in science and mathematics taken during high school provide intellectual challenge and difficult content and consequently require a greater and more intensive commitment of time from students. Individuals who had completed one or more of these courses successfully developed study habits that would contribute to their later success in a college premed curriculum. The persisters had taken more of these enhanced courses than their nonpersisting peers.

Persisters more often than nonpersisters took Algebra I before the ninth grade and took calculus while in high school. They earned higher grades, on average, in Algebra II and in trigonometry than the students who left premed, but too few nonpersisters took calculus for a grade comparison to be made. Persisters were pretty evenly divided between science and nonscience as the favorite course taken in the first year of college, while a strong majority of the nonpersisters interviewed chose a nonscience course. And persisters were somewhat more likely than nonpersisters to have included science or math as the favorite high school subject.

A finding somewhat difficult to account for is that among the 19 students who attended a single-sex high school, all but one were persisters. It may be that students in single-sex schools had less distraction during the school day and were able to develop good study habits, or it may be that these particular schools were different in some other way.

There were differences outside the classroom, too. Playing with science toys as a child did not differentiate the two groups, but the nonpersisters were less likely to understand machinery. Persisters were more likely than nonpersisters to have been highly committed to one or more out-of-class activities while in high school, but slightly more than half of the students in both groups had performed community service while in high school. The norm for both groups was to spend 5 hours or less on household chores and in caring for others on a weekly basis, but persisters were *more* likely (57% to 45%) to have been employed while in high school. The rate of high school employment was lower, however, than rates reported using national data (Manning, 1990). There was one interesting difference between the groups on dating frequency in high school: All those students who did not date in the tenth grade, eleventh, and twelfth grades were persisters.

In summary, persisters had better preparation in science, greater understanding of machines, and higher levels of commitment to an extracurricular activity in high school. Part-time employment did not impede their academic success.

Differences in the First Year of College

The higher performers in both semesters of general chemistry and in the accompanying labs were persisters, although their grades in these courses were not especially high. One-third of persisters earned grades of B or better in the first-semester course, compared with 20% of nonpersisters. Because general chemistry was the first filter for premeds, the students were asked about their preparation for that course, performance in the course, and behaviors associated with that performance. Nonpersisters were more likely to say that their class notes were *of no importance* when they studied for exams. Students who do not understand the material in the class lectures are less likely to take notes of high quality. They may take down only part of what the professor says or take notes that do not make sense when read later on.

Persisters were far more likely to be involved in one or more study groups for premed courses but did not spend more time studying and did not feel freer to ask questions in class. At the extreme, however, *all* those students who had always felt free to ask questions in their first-year premed classes persisted to the second year. Persisters were no less likely than nonpersisters to take verbatim notes, but nonpersisters were more likely to memorize material for exams while persisters attempted to understand the material. Most students (from both groups) did only *some* of the chemistry problems, and persisters were not more likely to do *all* of them.

Persisters were more likely to have selected medicine as their career prior to entering high school and hence had a longer-term investment in the goal of medical school. In their first year of college, they were no more likely to say that financial security and prosperity were important in their selection of a medical career, or to place higher value on respect from others, than were the nonpersisters. Interest in helping people was the most important factor selected by both groups.

The importance of the specific motivation to pursue medicine and its relation to persistence can be better understood with reference to grades. To what extent were premeds with lower levels of achievement still persisting, in part because of the attraction of high income later on? Students with grade-point averages lower than 3.00 are far less likely to be admitted to medical school. Those persisters with less than a 3.00 GPA in the first year were more interested in the financial rewards of medicine than were their peers with higher grades. There is no other occupation that yields such high financial rewards, on average, so some premeds who are attracted for this reason will persist until they have no hope of succeeding.

Those premeds with lower grades who valued only altruism among the three types of rewards would be expected to leave the premed program to pursue other career options where they could do good for others. Instead, they demonstrated strong attachment to medicine as the specific vehicle for doing good. An early decision to be a doctor, combined with the hope of someday being in a position to save lives, was strong enough motivation for them to continue, despite the odds against their success. Yet even some very good students, strongly motivated by the altruistic aspect of medicine, questioned their career choice. One student, with better than a 3.50 GPA, expressed it this way: "I have thought about social work. That would allow me to work with and help people but is not related to my performance in premed courses."

While a majority of persisters and nonpersisters reported having received peer support in high school for the study of math and science, nonpersisters had received *more* support from peers and *more* support from their parents for continuing in math and science while in high school. Persisters were more likely to say that they did not discuss curriculum issues with their parents. In college, however, it was the persisters who were more likely to say that they received moderate or strong support from their peers for continuing in premed. Some of the nonpersisters may have entered premed initially not because of an interest or ability in science or a personal preference for medicine, but because of parental encouragement they received for pursuing science and medicine. This interpretation is strengthened by the reasons given for valuing success in premed courses. Nonpersisters were more likely to say that success in difficult endeavors demonstrates competence and provides self-esteem; when the self-esteem rewards decline, the reason to persist also diminishes.

Persisters perceived that they were doing relatively better than other students, although their grades may not have been As. The subjective assessments of their performance vis à vis other students in the class accurately reflected their earned grades in these courses, even though they made their assessments before final grades were assigned. While they would not have known the actual grades of many of the other students in their classes, they were able to recognize a range in performance. If they saw themselves as the poor performers, they assigned themselves the lower subjective rankings; if others were the poor performers, they assigned themselves the *better-than-average* rankings, even though their actual numerical or letter grade at that time was not especially high. Because of the practice of grading on the curve, they could assume that their final grade would be at least in the top half of the distribution. Persisters outperformed nonpersisters on grade-point average at the close of the first year by 2.94 to 2.57.

PERSISTING AFTER THE SECOND YEAR

Students who enrolled in a premed course for the junior year and students who had completed premed requirements at the close of the sophomore year were included as persisting through time 2. Interview data on nonpersisters are more limited than for persisters, especially from the second and last interviews. Some reference will be made to comparisons on background factors and to first-year experience, when they impact on staying and leaving after the second year.

Those still in premed were more likely to have decided on medicine early, before starting high school. While many high school experiences would not be expected to have an impact on behavior after 2 years of college, a stronger or weaker academic foundation, especially in math and science, can have a long-term impact. Persisters at this point were more likely than nonpersisters to have taken physics and a second year of chemistry while in high school. And persisters were more likely to have earned As in those science courses that most of them completed in high school: Biology I and II, Chemistry I, and Physics I. It is not surprising that those who would persist through 2 years of premed were far more likely to earn B or better grades in general chemistry and general biology courses in college. GPA overall after the second year of college favored persisters, 3.05 versus 2.75. This average level of performance (of persisters) still was not competitive for medical school admission, another reminder that staying in premed and progressing toward medical school were not necessarily synonymous.

At the close of the second year, the nonpersisters' interest in science had declined to the point that *not one* of them chose a science course as their favorite. Persisters and nonpersisters alike chose a favorite course based on its subject matter—science for the former, something else for the latter. Persisters were more likely to have joined study groups for premed courses. While more than half of the persons in each group felt free to ask questions in class at least sometimes, persisters were more likely to say that they always felt free to do so. The nonpersisters were more likely during each of the first 2 years to memorize material rather than attempt to understand it. By the end of the second year of college, the primary distinction between the two groups was science—interest in, love of, and often a demonstrated ability in it for the persisters and the absence of all these for the nonpersisters. Even those remaining in premed had complaints, however: large classes, incomprehensible lectures, and professors who seemed to expect scientific genius in their undergraduate students. Yet most persisters had discovered that science was interesting and, for a growing number, relevant to medicine.

There was very little difference in the education of mothers or fathers of students who persisted in premed through the second year and those who did not. Fathers overwhelmingly were employed in professional and managerial occupations. Mothers of persisters were more likely to be in those occupations, too, while mothers of nonpersisters were most often found in technical and sales occupations. Contrary to any hypothesis of upward mobility—parents promoting medicine for their sons and especially daughters to improve their status and income levels—these data suggest that for most students the decision to pursue medicine had other motivation. Family income of persisters was higher, on average, than that of nonpersisters, a finding that may be explained in part by the difference in mother's occupation. The influence of a parent who was also a physician had declined by the end of the second year, with the children of physicians nearly equally represented among persisters and nonpersisters. While the influence or support from a physician-parent may have contributed significantly to some of these students having an early interest in medicine, for some the interest could not be sustained though the rigorous premed curriculum.

While nonpersisters were more likely to report having a doctor in their family, this inverse relationship is not as surprising as it first appears. Some students reported being discouraged from the pursuit of medicine by family members and friends in the medical profession, who saw medicine changing in undesirable ways. If premed students did not derive their commitment from personal passion at this stage, they were more likely to listen to such pessimistic predictions. Some were attracted to medicine initially after watching a family member practice and only later, after performing less well than expected in required courses, became nonpersisters.

There was some relationship between demographic characteristics and persistence. Birth order had limited relationship to persistence, except among *only* children, 93% of whom continued in premed into the third year. Women stayed in premed at a higher rate than men; 81% of the women still at the university and 71% of the men were premed in the third year. The highest persistence rates by racial/ethnic group were found among the Asian Americans (95%) and African Americans (82%). The sole Native American student, too, was a persister. The persistence rates among non-Hispanic whites was 73% and among Hispanic premeds, 57%.

There was some consensus among the persisters on the attractions of medicine to them: interest in helping people and intellectual challenge. Nonpersisters, on the other hand, agreed only on their desire to help people. Money and respect from others, like altruism, were no more likely to be regarded as important by one group than by the other.

PERSISTING INTO THE FOURTH YEAR

Included among the nonpersisters at each time period were individuals who had left premed at any time since the study began, so long as they were still enrolled in the institution. Persons who left the university were not included in either group. The definition of persister used at time 3 was more restrictive than some of these premeds would have liked. Persisters at time 3 were premeds who had taken the MCAT at least once and applied to one or more medical schools within a year of finishing college. Since most persons entering a premed program in their first year of college hoped to enter medical school 4 years later, those who were not prepared to take the MCAT or not ready for medical school within a year after graduating were regarded as nonpersisters. While some of these men and women would apply in a later year, many of them had not applied yet because their grades or scores were not competitive. Of the 131 individuals included in the analysis at time 3, 52 were classified as persisters and 79 as nonpersisters.

The academic success of persisters in comparison with nonpersisters is the factor that was least in doubt. The premeds with lower grades were likely to have left the program. The courses and grades that contributed to persistence at earlier stages continued to do so. Yet the persisters at time 3 had to do more than complete courses satisfactorily. They also had to take action—by signing up for and taking the MCAT and applying to at least one medical school. College grades in required courses and overall GPA (3.37 versus 2.81) favored the persisters by a wide margin. Since few nonpersisters took the MCAT, the discussion will shift somewhat to persisters and to premeds accepted to medical school.

GPA is both cause and consequence of persistence. Students earning high grades were motivated to persist, and students interested in science who went on to take advanced courses in science were likely to improve their grades. By the second semester of the senior year, when the third interview was conducted, MCAT scores had been received and were another objective measure of performance. If a student did not take the MCAT, it was because he or she feared not doing well or was ambivalent about medicine. Some of the test-takers received low scores and attributed their performance to mitigating factors—a heavy course load that semester that left too little time for preparation, illness, personal or family problems at that time, or a lack of effort. The knowledge that their performance as measured by national norms was unsatisfactory would increase the pressure when taking the exam a second time. Their earlier performance was poor, and the distribution of scores nationally is such that they would need to score well above the midpoint to be competitive—even higher for those medical schools that average the two scores instead of using only the best or most recent test. These premeds had to decide whether to work toward the goal for another year or not.

Students who were not discouraged upon receipt of their MCAT scores (and even some who were) made formal application to medical schools at the end of the junior year. There was little to decide at this point if the scores were at least average, for while the application process is long and taxing, only a loss of interest (or the substitution of a new interest) and the cost of applying are obvious deterrents. Even cost was not likely to prevent interested students from applying to a small number of schools in the state where they lived or attended college.

Most of the persisters took the MCAT late in the spring of their third year. As discussed in Chapter 2, scores on this day-long test of four parts—verbal reasoning, biological sciences, physical sciences (all multiple-choice), and essay—have a significant impact on the decision to admit or not to admit an applicant. Consequently, it is a test that few takers regard casually. Mean scores on the subtests for *all* test-takers in 1993 were 7.68 on verbal reasoning, 7.87 on biological sciences, and 7.73 on physical sciences (AAMC, 1994a). The mean verbal subtest score on the MCAT for the premeds in my sample was 8.7; the highest verbal score was 14 (of a possible 15). The mean on the biological sciences subtest was 8.4, with a high of 13. On the physical sciences subtest, the mean score was 8.1 and the highest score was 13. The scores of this small population of 52 test-takers were affected somewhat by the lower scores of some students for whom English was not the first language.

This population of test-takers was self-selected. Because anyone completing the prerequisite courses could be premed, even with low grades in required courses, and thus could take the MCAT, test averages for all applicants are not very informative. More instructive for premeds who hope to be accepted are the mean scores of students from this sample who were subsequently admitted to a medical school: 9.4 verbal, 8.7 biological sciences, and 8.4 physical sciences. Most students at the time of the third interview had taken the MCAT only once. When multiple scores were available for a student, only the higher score was coded. Depending on the date of their decision to accept or reject, medical schools may have had more recent scores available or may have used a different method of assigning weights to the two sets of scores.

Research on gender differences on standardized test scores has found that "the SAT underpredicts the performance of women in college, including in courses in science and mathematics" (Betz, 1994, p. 241). MCAT results show that men outperform women, on average, on the science subtests and that women do not necessarily outperform men on the verbal subtest. It is important not to overstate the difference, however, since the distributions of scores overlap—some women earn high scores and some men earn low scores. Test anxiety, more prevalent among women than among men, may contribute to these gender differences in MCAT scores. There is a great deal resting on performance on this test, which is given only twice each year. Individuals who take the test in late summer will have complete applications to present to medical schools only after the school has already received many times the number of qualified applicants needed to fill the next class. Persons who apply early receive earlier consideration. A study of applicants to one medical school documented that those who applied and were considered early were more likely to be accepted for that year than later applicants. The exception was out-of-state applicants to state medical schools (Elam & Johnson, 1997a). Consequently, the chances of admission for the year following college graduation rest for most applicants on a test taken only once.

In 1993, 56% of MCAT examinees nationally were men and 44%, women. Men outperformed women on the 1993 MCAT—slightly on the verbal (7.70 versus 7.65) and more decisively on the biological science (8.19 versus 7.46) and physical science (8.20 versus 7.14) subtests. Women earned higher scores than men on the essay (AAMC, 1994a, pp. 27, 63). These scores are the means for the population of test-takers that year; test averages for applicants and entrants to medical school will be higher. The MCAT scores of the men and women in the premed sample were 8.9 (men) and 8.5 (women) on the verbal subtest; 8.8 (men) and 8.2 (women) on biological sciences; and 8.4 (men) and 8.0 (women) on physical sciences. While gender comparisons on standardized tests usually favor males, in this sample the scores of women were depressed more than those of men by a higher proportion of women whose first language was not English. Taking this into consideration, the differences reflect more than gender.

GENDER DIFFERENCES

One of the significant changes in patterns of application and acceptance to medical schools has been in gender composition. Yet, while more women are applying and being accepted than in the past, differences between men and women remain.

Persistence

Women were accepted to a coeducational medical school for the first time in 1849–50, comprising 3% of the entering class at the Central Medical College of New York at Syracuse (Lopate, 1968). It is only recently that the percentage of women applying to and enrolling in medical schools has approached, equaled, and in some cases exceeded that of men. As noted in Chapter 2, one study of admission to U.S. medical schools found that from 1929 to 1984 women were accepted in roughly the same ratio of acceptances-to-applications as men, when the school accepted women at all (Cole, 1986). Forty-eight percent of women who applied in 1964–65 were accepted, compared with 47% of men, yet ten times as many men as women applied (Lopate, 1968). Commenting on the entering class of 1991, Plantz and colleagues (1993) noted: "Of 13,700 female applicants, 6,433, or 46.9%, were accepted. This compares to 19,601 male applicants with 10,493 accepted, or 53.5%" (p. 118). Women comprised more than half of the entering classes in fall 1994 of Harvard, Yale, Johns Hopkins, and 15 other medical schools, and they comprised 42% of new students in U.S. medical schools overall ("Women Increasing," 1995, p. A9).

   Fiorentine and Cole (1992) found that men and women entered *premed* programs in roughly equal ratios to their enrollment in college, yet men were "twice as likely to complete the program and apply to medical school" (p. 471). They noted the influence of GPA on the decision to stay or to leave: "Females with a . . . grade-point average of 3.50 or higher are no less likely to persist in the program and apply to medical school" (p. 471). Those women whose grades were high enough to merit possible consideration but not high enough to make them feel confident that they would be admitted, with GPAs in the 3.00–3.50 range, had to decide whether the costs involved in preparing for medicine—the time, effort, and anxiety—would be worth the return. Fiorentine (1988) concluded from the same study that "to a student struggling in one of the most competitive majors on campus, with nearly a decade of training ahead, even slight doubts about his or her ability could tip the balance from persistence to defection" (p. 243). Men were more likely to persist "until they experience almost no possibility of success" and women "only until there is some reasonable possibility of failure" (p. 247).

The choice of a nontraditional career is still a difficult one for some women, especially those who have less social support for their choice. Carney and Morgan (1981) found that among college seniors,

> women in non-traditional major fields were found to have higher ACT scores, . . . higher degree expectations, to feel better prepared in math, to have higher grades in high school math, to come from higher family income levels, [and] to view women's roles outside the home as less restrictive than [did] women in traditional fields of study. (p. 420)

With reduced structural and cultural constraints on women wishing to enter medicine today, persistence now is affected less by gender per se and more by the depth of motivation to become a doctor and the number of attractive occupational alternatives available. If an individual wants to serve humankind above all else, by maintaining or restoring health in others, the fields of public health, social work, and nursing are among the alternatives to medicine. If the professional interest extends beyond the health fields, education can be added to this list of service professions. If autonomy, social recognition, and financial security are also desired or necessary criteria for an occupation, then individuals are most likely to stay in (pre)medicine "until they experience almost no possibility of success."

The women persisters chose medicine as their goal earlier, on average, than the men, and were more likely to have taken advanced math and science courses in high school. More than men, they took Biology II (but not Chemistry II) in high school, Algebra I in junior high, and calculus before college. To the extent that understanding machinery contributed to success in science classes, the advantage went to the men, more of whom claimed to have at least a moderate understanding. The men also were more likely than the women to have committed themselves at the highest level to an activity throughout high school.

While most of the *only* children were persisters, most of them were also women. Likewise with oldest children—a majority persisted through the second year, and a majority of them were women. The advantages of parents' education, income, and elder/only child status resulted in some advantages for these women premeds that would not necessarily be found in other populations of college students. Yet there is evidence here that the effects of gender per se have lessened. The social and cultural capital that parents have to pass on to their children in the form of enriched home and school environments, wealth, contacts, and opportunities—capital that once was passed on only to sons—now goes to daughters as well. Women more often than men said that their parents supported them a great deal in their study of math and science while in high school and in the premed program once in college. It was not likely that parents were indifferent to their sons' progress in meeting their goals. It is more likely that parents of premed daughters saw greater need for providing support for success in a male-dominated profession. A study of students in medical school found that "significantly more women students (85%) than men students (70%) said they had . . . support for their career decision" (Kutner & Brogan, 1980, p. 351).

Once in college, gender differences between these persisters diminished but did not disappear. While a majority of persisting women and men earned grades of B or better in General Biology, men were far more likely to earn As in this course. But the women outperformed the men in General Chemistry I and II and also in organic chemistry, where a higher percentage of women than men earned As. Men were more likely to belong to study groups but no more likely to feel free to ask questions in class. Women in our sample were more likely than men to persist in premed into the fourth year—33 of the 76 women (43%) from the original sample who were still enrolled in the university and 19 of 55 of the men (35%). In the fourth year, men submitted nine applications to medical schools, on average, and women, seven. Although the men earned higher MCAT scores, cumulative GPA at that time favored the women, 3.09 versus 2.95 for the men.

The premed women entered college with math and science preparation, SAT scores, and social support equal to or greater than that of the men, and women stayed in premed in a higher proportion than men. Women recognized that they were doing well, using their classmates as their reference group. Yet women in their interviews more often than men were ambivalent about having careers in medicine, apprehensive about its time demands and its tendency to reduce other aspects of life to secondary importance. Despite support and grades competitive with men and the same expected marriage age for both, women were more likely to have questioned their career goals during the first 2 years. So, while the academic record of these women predicted an eventual acceptance to medical school at a rate at least equal to that for men, women were more likely to express reservations about medicine.

Attitudes Toward Career and Family

This study began with the assumption that men and women premeds would differ somewhat in their views on life and work. That those differences are not as great as they once were should not lead to the conclusion that they have disappeared. Men were less likely than women to fear social stigma from working *too much* once they had launched a professional career or to be concerned about the impact of their professional choice on their personal relationships. While the popular press and the medical and psychological literature on stress and its consequences are changing our collective perception of the value of spending unlimited hours at work, there is still a gender effect. The combined aspirations for career and family introduced stress for premeds who recognized the potential conflict. This stress was experienced far more often by women than by men. One woman in our study expressed these concerns more immediately, since she was planning to get married very soon. Other women saw the competing demands for time and attention converging within the next several years:

> I don't think medicine is my calling. I don't want to stay in school 7 more years and work as hard as I have worked, with so little benefit. I want a family.

> Now I know I want marriage and a family. Then [when she started the premed program], I thought my career would be everything.

> I have selected dermatology [as my medical specialty] because I can schedule work around the demands of family and marriage later on.

A few women shifted their interest from medicine to dentistry, which they saw as offering them more time and greater independence:

> I've realized that I want more than a career; I want a family and I want time for myself. I've begun to think of dentistry as an alternative to medicine.

> The whole health care reform is frightening, taking out loans for medical school but not knowing how medicine will change. There are many other things I want to do in my life. Medicine requires that you be a doctor 24 hours a day. I want some autonomy, in a small [dental] practice.

And there was a different view: "Most of my friends and I share the same goals: We want to be more than mothers." It is noteworthy that these comments and others like them came only from women. During the first year of college, plans for the future were still quite tentative for most of the respondents. By the fourth year, 95% of persisting men and 90% of persisting women expected to marry—at age 27, on average. While it might have been expected that premed students would delay marriage longer than these data suggest, Katchadourian and Boli (1994), in their study of Stanford graduates, noted:

> The timing of marriage does not seem to be affected much by type of professional preparation; future doctors have the longest road to travel, but they were almost as likely (23%) to be married by the fifth year (after graduation) as the average respondent. (p. 181)

In the interviews for our study, marriage was undefined and some of the respondents may have had in mind a long-term commitment to a partner of either sex rather than a more traditional marriage. Eighty-eight percent of men and all the women wanted to have children. The age chosen to start a family was 30, for both women and men; many respondents, however, did not have a specific age in mind.

For most college-educated women today it is difficult if not impossible to select career *or* family as having higher priority. Instead, it is the challenge of combining career *and* family that is the highest priority. The importance of career success and financial rewards among personal goals of college women nationwide has been increasing. When the participants in our study were in their first or second year of college, college freshman women nationwide listed among their objectives becoming an authority in their field (64%) and being well-off financially (70%) (Astin, 1990, p. A31). These data compare with those from 1969, when 54% of college freshman women wanted to be an authority in their field, and those from 1971, when being well off financially was important to only 28% of women (American Council on Education data, cited by Fiorentine, 1988a, p. 148).

APPLICATION AND ACCEPTANCE

A subset of the persisters were those premeds who attained their goal of admission to a medical school. They are the focus of this section.

Premeds whose success in this lengthy process included multiple acceptances to medical school could approximate a rational decision-making strategy. There were usually weeks or even months before having to make a final choice and hence time to gather relevant information on the choice alternatives. With few exceptions, they had visited the schools, so they had some knowledge of facilities, familiarity with the area surrounding each school, and some limited contact with current students. Information about financial aid, housing, curriculum, and clinical experience was available from the schools. In comparison with some other life decisions, the relevant information available to these premed decision makers was abundant. Although there are some differences in emphases across schools, and only some institutions offered the MD/PhD programs that were the goal of a few premeds, there is relatively little risk of making a *bad* choice in selecting a U.S. medical school. They are accredited similarly, their faculties possess similar educational qualifications, and fellow students were high achievers in their respective colleges. Requirements for accreditation eliminate the possibility of a below-standard medical education.

"Slightly less than half (48.4%) of the applicants to U.S. MD-granting institutions for entrance in 1992 received two or more acceptances" (Corder, 1994, p. 65). For the class entering medical school in 1993, "the 16,500 places being offered this year are about the same number that have been offered since 1980. . . . The average medical school applicant applies to 11 medical schools" (Altman, 1993, p. A10). Most schools participate in AM-CAS, the American College Application Service. AMCAS assists the applicants, for a fee, by disseminating to medical schools the academic information and other material supplied by the applicants. AMCAS assists the medical schools even more, providing each applicant's material in a standard format and verifying the accuracy of academic information and MCAT scores. With only 127 medical schools in the United States, a single student may apply to even 15% of them. One school in 1994 had received 10,000 applications for its 150 places, a ratio of 67 applicants for each space. The same school 30 years earlier had 8 applicants per space (Bloom, 1973, p. 33). So, while aspirants are advised while in college to apply to many schools, the fact remains that only one in three of those men and women making application will be informed that they have a seat in next year's class. And over 60% of applicants will not be admitted.

At the time of the final data collection for this study, in the spring of the senior year, only one of the study participants was already in medical school, having been accepted through an early-admission program. The 52 premed persisters submitted an average of 8 applications; the range was 2 to 20. Because their university kept records of acceptances, a small number of premeds were included in the data on applicants who had not been accepted on their first attempt but were accepted for the next year. By the second year after graduation, 40 of the 52 had been accepted, including one applicant accepted to a DO program. Another individual was accepted the following year. Two among the total were accepted to schools outside the United States. These acceptance data exclude four students who were

TABLE 5.1. Performance Measures (Mean Values) for Accepted Students

Pre-College

Took calculus in high school	67%
Grade in calculus	A-
Cumulative GPA	3.71
Best SAT score	
Verbal	615
Math	624

College

Science Grades	
General Biology I*	B+
General Chemistry I & II	B
Physics I & II	B+
Organic Chemistry I & II	B
Cumulative GPA	
After year 1	3.37
After year 2	3.45
After year 3	3.49
*MCAT scores**	
Verbal	9.4
Biological science	8.7
Physical science	8.4

*Grades in the second (required) biology course were not included, as premeds chose from among several alternative courses to satisfy this requirement.
**MCAT scores shown here do not take into account retests after the last interview. Premeds who were accepted a year later may have had higher scores than those included in these counts, raising the average slightly for the group as a whole.

admitted to dental schools only. Two additional participants in this study, both women, were admitted to one or more medical schools, but they had not been classified as persisters at time 3. They had decided against medicine, left the study, and then changed their minds while still in college. Adding them to the persisters, the acceptance rate increases to 80%, with most of the successful applicants receiving one or two acceptances. The magnitude of the competition can surprise even applicants with stronger qualifications: "I thought I'd get into a lot more medical schools".

Data on the accepted premeds are presented in Tables 5.1 through 5.4, grouped into categories of variables used throughout the book: performance and related behaviors, motivation, and support. Table 5.1 shows the mean value of performance measures in high school and college for the accepted premeds. Contributing to each of these averages is a range of values. It was not uncommon in each of the required premed courses to find one or more students with C grades. There were a few grades lower than C, too. This was evidence that a single poor grade in a required course, when placed in the context of a stronger overall record, does not *necessarily* keep an individual out of medical school.

When asked to evaluate their performance in required courses in comparison with their peers, from "one of the best" to "one of the worst" in the class, most of these accepted medical students evaluated themselves favorably, as "better than many in the class." Yet there was no one-to-one relationship between the grade earned in the course and the subjective assessment of performance. Using General Chemistry I as an example, only those students confident enough to describe their performance as *one of the best in the class* were accurate. Five persons described their performance as *best*, and all five earned A or A– grades. The range was widest for the *better than many* response, chosen by 19 individuals whose grades in the course were distributed evenly across A, B+, B, and B– levels, and one recipient of a C+ grade. Such inexact matches reflected uncertainty about the level of achievement in courses using norm-referenced grading. When asked to assess their performance in General Chemistry I, they already knew their letter grade in the course. In all of the premed science courses and cumulatively, premeds accepted to medical school outperformed persisters overall. It was evident that understanding machinery was not necessary for success in premed or for entrance to medical school, since many respondents reported having virtually no such understanding.

Table 5.2 highlights some behaviors that contributed to academic success. From the first to the second year there was a decrease in the size of the majority studying to understand, yet most of the others said that they combined the two strategies of memorizing and understanding, so they, too, *studied to understand*. The range in the number of hours spent studying is worth comment: in year 1 one person spent 6 hours a week and another 65 hours, the low and high points of this distribution. In year 2, the range was narrower, 12 to 50 hours. By year 4 the range was 3 to 90 hours, the latter from a student working on a particularly demanding honors thesis. When his data were excluded, the group average declined from 27 to 25 hours a week.

Differences in behaviors were small between the larger group of those who persisted and those who were admitted. The largest was a difference of only 7 percentage points, in favor of persisters, in the number belonging

TABLE 5.2. Behavior Measures for Accepted Students

Pre-College

Hours/week spent on household chores or the care of others[a]	6
Number of enhanced or advanced math and science courses[a]	3
Committed to an activity 5+ hours/week for 4 years	51%

College

In study groups in year 1	38%
Did all problems in General Chemistry I	28%
Had contact with premed adviser in year 1	65%
Studied to understand	
in year 1	73%
in year 2	57%
Studied throughout the term	75%
Hours/week studied	
in year 1[a]	24
in year 2[a]	26
in year 4[a]	27
Number of medical schools applied to[a]	7

[a]Mean value

to study groups—38% of accepted students versus 46% for persisters over-all.

As shown in Table 5.3, financial rewards were not important to a majority of the accepted students, and social rewards declined in importance during the undergraduate years. In contrast, a strong interest in science and the desire to help others sustained their interest in the intrinsic rewards of medicine. The valued rewards from medicine were similar for accepted students and for persisters generally. Among the few notable differences between the two groups were the greater importance of school rank to accepted students in year 1 and more persisters selecting science as their favorite course in year 1. Two-thirds of the accepted students had majored in biology.

The data in Table 5.4 show that premeds were most likely to report receiving moderate or strong support from their high school teachers or counselor. Perhaps their support was more memorable than that received

TABLE 5.3. Motivation Measures for Accepted Students

Pre-College

Decided on medicine pre-high school	56%
Favorite high school subject was biology	42%

College

Academic interest

Biology (when entering college)	61%
Science/math favorite course year 1	46%
Science interest same or increased years 1-4	97%

Importance of rewards

Financial	
year 1	46%
year 4	42%
Social	
year 1	76%
year 4	67%
Altruism	
year 1	100%
year 4	100%

TABLE 5.4. Social Support Measures for Accepted Students

Pre-College

Encouragement For Science/Math Moderate/Strong:

From parents	54%
From high school peers	62%
From teachers or counselor	89%

College

Support For Remaining In Premed Moderate/Strong:

From parents	78%
From peers	69%

from parents or peers because it was more likely to focus on specific events, such as the selection of high school courses or college applications. Parents' support was higher for remaining in premed than it was earlier, for taking math and science courses. Data for persisters, in comparison with these data for accepted students, show parents' support at 50%, high school peers' support at 58%, teachers'/counselor's support at 90%, and college peers' support at 73%, very similar to the profile of the accepted students.

In spite of the superior or equal performance of women in many of the required science courses, and their higher grades overall, women in this sample were far less likely to get into medical school than their male peers, with 71% of the women applicants and 95% of the men accepted. Explanation for this difference rests in part with grades and scores. Four of ten women who had not received acceptances, but not the one man, had cumulative grade-point averages at the time of application below 3.00. All of the women who had not been accepted, and the man, had MCAT totals below 27, averaging less than 9 for each subtest. And women applied to fewer schools, on average, than men. Another gender difference is that two men, but no women, applied to and were accepted to medical schools outside the United States, where admission was less competitive.

There could have been a self-selection factor that was different for men and women, although the direction of this effect is against what might have been expected, based on the research on persistence in math- and science-related programs. While past research has shown that women are less likely than men to continue working toward a goal when the chance of success is low, the results from this study show that women with lower MCAT scores still applied to medical school. Some of the gender difference may be explained by another difference between the two samples: There were more women than men who were foreign-born or who were members of underrepresented minority groups. If more of these individuals than in the other groups in the sample saw medicine or had parents who saw medicine as upward mobility, these premeds may have been less willing to give up on their goal, even if their MCAT scores or grades were lower than the average for accepted students. While one study does not indicate social change, it should not be surprising that women who have been encouraged in their educational and occupational aspirations and who have worked toward a goal over a number of years would pursue it to the end—until reaching it or until further progress is blocked.

The accepted population was 60% non-Hispanic white, 21% Asian American, and 19% underrepresented minorities. This translates into acceptance rates for the three racial groups as follows: 81% of non-Hispanic whites who applied were accepted, compared with 75% of Asian Americans and 80% of underrepresented minorities.

Some background factors, especially socioeconomic status (SES), were used in comparing accepted students with persisters. Fathers' and mothers' education was lower among accepted students than among persisters generally. Fathers' and mothers' occupational status, too, was lower among accepted premeds. Contrary to the beliefs of a few of the study participants, children of physician parents were not more likely to be admitted, although that may have been a factor in some individual cases. Accepted premeds were not more likely than persisters generally to have high family incomes. These data contrast with those of an earlier study, when Leserman (1981) noted that "the children of the working classes are less likely to achieve the privileged status of physician" (p. 83).

PERSISTENCE BEYOND COLLEGE

Some premeds in the study decided to delay their application, until the next year or indefinitely, for various reasons. For some, *later* was a preferable interview response to not applying. *Later* reflects uncertainty of one kind or another—doubts about the desirability of medicine as a career, especially in the context of the national conversation about health care going on at that time, or fear that one's MCAT scores and grades will not be high enough to gain admission.

Individuals who are rejected on the first try cannot expect the competition to lessen in the next year. Yet applicants do try again. According to Kassebaum and Szenas (1995), the size of the applicant pool increased significantly between 1988 and 1994, with repeat applicants contributing disproportionally more to the increase than first-time applicants. These authors noted that the increase in the applicant pool corresponded to a leaner job market for college graduates. Some premeds in this study did improve their MCAT scores significantly on the second try, and others distinguished themselves in a graduate program. Just persisting, reapplying without a solid strategy for improving relative standing in the next year's pool, is not sufficient.

To understand the nature and strength of motivation to pursue medicine, it is helpful to look at some individuals whose aspirations changed or were delayed. Colquitt and Killian (1991) reported on a group surveyed by the Association of American Medical Colleges who took the MCAT but had not applied to medical school. At the time of taking the exam, they intended to apply to one or more schools and their MCAT scores at least approached the mean. "The most frequent dissuading factor, reported by 48%, was . . . [that] 'physicians with whom I have counseled have not been encouraging about the future of medicine'" (p. 276). While that reaction was not commonly reported by our students, at least one had encountered it:

> I don't like the attitude of many doctors who told me "you won't make as much money in the future; don't be a doctor." They have lost the ability to relate to people who aren't white-collar.

Another student said that his family did not encourage him to be a doctor, although his father was a doctor.

Because of the lengthy period between their initial choice of medicine and the time when they learn whether they have been accepted for next year's medical school class, those who persist all the way through college have a difficult time letting go if they are not admitted on their first attempt. One study of 98 men and women rejected by all medical schools to which they had applied found that 12 eventually were admitted. The women who persisted and continued to reapply after rejection were those who were most interested in science (Radius, Becker, Smith, & Katatsky, 1979). Applicants who are rejected the first time will not be admitted on a subsequent try unless they improve their qualifications significantly. *Beginning* a graduate program will not help in subsequently gaining admission to medical school; successfully completing the program might help. Some, however, hope that sheer determination will be convincing:

> I plan to keep applying until I get in, unless it's 5 years or so from now; then I may have to change directions.

> I want to go to medical school. I'll go to Grenada if I have to.

> I've thought that if I don't get into medical school this year, I'll go to graduate school and reapply. I'm set on becoming a doctor.

Another segment of the applicant pool consists of individuals who are older but applying for the first time. While approximately 40% of the applicant pool consists of persons 24 years of age and older (Ramsbottom-Lucier, Johnson, & Elam, 1995), many of these applicants are only 2 to 3 years out of college. Some deferred college, and others had interruptions in their college programs; they are not likely to be very different from other applicants. The rest are persons who turned to medicine after beginning another career. Their applications are more easily distinguished from the rest of the applicant pool. Admissions committees may decide that individuals from this population add maturity and a different perspective to the class, increasing the probability of acceptance for those whose grades and scores are also acceptable.

In some graduate programs outside medicine, first-year students are aware that some members of their cohort might not be retained for a second year, following a qualifying exam or review of their first-year performance by the faculty. Criteria for retention are not always well understood by students. Medical school provides a notable contrast. Admission to a medical school is the big hurdle for prospective doctors, and a large majority of those admitted are retained. This fact, too, adds to an applicant's reasons for persisting after rejection.

SUMMARIZING THE EXPERIENCE

In summary, comparisons at each stage between those premeds who persisted in their preparation for medical school and those who did not show some differences in background factors, in gender, in behavior and performance, in support, and in motivation. While persistence is affected primarily by more recent factors, the effects of performance, in particular, are cumulative, measured in the longer term. It is not only the grades in the recent courses and the cumulative GPA that are taken into consideration, but grades overall and grades in science courses, even those taken early in college. The encouraging news for all current and aspiring premeds is that a single disappointing performance in a science course by itself is insufficient to close the door to medical school. Yet the acceptance rate for women in this sample, who persisted in greater proportion than the men, lagged far behind that of the men. While some of this difference was attributable to MCAT scores and to factors peculiar to this sample, this gap is disturbing.

PREMED BIOGRAPHIES IN THE LAST YEAR

Most of the ten premeds profiled in this book applied to one or more medical schools during their senior year of college. Following the application was a period of waiting and then the result—an acceptance or a rejection. A variety of decisions and outcomes is exhibited among these men and women.

In spite of his A– cumulative grade-point average at the close of his third year and his high total score of 31 on the MCAT (on a scale of 0–45), *Michael* said that he questioned his career goals "at least once a semester. The overall stress level gets overwhelming." He was still employed part-time and volunteered at a hospital to increase his exposure to medicine. As he approached graduation, he said that his friends were "putting him down" because he still had so many years of schooling to complete. His response: "I think those who work hard will do better later, at least I hope so." When asked about positive aspects of the premed experience, Michael mentioned the respect that he received from other students and from adults. The negative—having *no* social life. "I had one night a week at best to goof off." He described an upper-level biology course as the most difficult course he had taken in college: "the most phenomenal amount of information I have ever had to know." Constructive study habits were an asset for Michael, who entered college having already developed the discipline to put his studies first. And it paid off for him; he was accepted to three medical schools.

Emily, too, named an upper-level biology course as her most difficult: "It was boring and required lab work that I did not enjoy. It was hard to study for, because I hated it." Yet she "loved" biochemistry. When asked about her views on medicine as a career for her, Emily said "I have thought more seriously about medical school affecting my personal life, especially as a woman. The competition has gotten to me and I have lost friendships over borrowed class notes. Premeds are really cut-throat." She questioned her career goals "every day." "The whole thing is a hazing process, through the residency. What is the point? This process is responsible in part for doctors' expecting so much when they get out." Emily began the application process, then withdrew her applications after receiving her MCAT scores, which totaled less than 25. She planned to reapply the next year. She, like Michael, expressed concerns about the impact of premed and medical school on social life. "I have concerns about having a life beyond school; I am not sure I can do this in medical school." All three attractions of medicine—the financial, social, and altruistic—were important to Emily.

Marsha decided while conducting research for her honors thesis that she wanted to pursue a combined MD/PhD program. When asked about the positive and negative aspects of her premed experience, she described the competition as something she enjoyed. The application process was confusing and, therefore, negative. She said that the altruistic and the financial rewards of medicine were important to her. With a cumulative grade-point average of 3.75 after 3 years and an MCAT score of 27, Marsha was accepted into a joint degree program.

In his senior year, *Ben* reported that Organic Chemistry II remained his most difficult course in college. He said that his interest in science had increased during the past year. "The more I got into it, . . . the more I understood and liked it." By his senior year, he had "no doubt" that he wanted to be a doctor. Reflecting on medicine, he said: "Doctors used to seem godlike; I now realize they have tough decisions to make and maybe don't know everything. I don't understand the costs—why are they so high?

I can't figure out where the money goes." All three rewards of medicine—the financial, altruistic, and social—were important to him. Having earned a very high score of 33 on the MCAT and an A– GPA, Ben was accepted to two of the medical schools to which he applied.

Amy dropped Organic Chemistry II in her third year. Referring to the volume of material and the pace of the course, she said it was the worst course she had ever taken. She decided against medicine soon afterwards, after taking the MCAT. She took her first course in business and "really enjoyed it." She went on to say, "It's like I found what I was supposed to do all along. . . . I am glad that I went through premed, because I tried it and realize it is not what I want. If I hadn't tried, I might have wished that I had. Now I know what I want and I am pleased with my decision."

Charles described how his interest in science had increased: "I see how the classes I have taken will help me in medical school." In each of the three interviews, he said that only the altruistic rewards of medicine were important to him, not the financial and social rewards. When asked how his views on medicine as a career for him had changed, he responded: "Premed used to be the thing to say" (i.e., it was a highly regarded choice), "but I have seen that medicine is not as glamorous as it is made out to be." Summing up what he had learned thus far about the practice of medicine, he said "doctors have to go through a lot." Charles earned just under a 3.4 GPA, applied to 11 schools, and received 3 acceptances.

In her senior year *Nora* still was not attracted to medicine because of its financial and social rewards but was very interested in helping others. She was a biology major and said that her interest in science had increased during the past year because of the difference between upper- and lower-level courses. "You learn more in the upper-level courses; the earlier courses were 'weed-out' courses." Nora's MCAT scores totaled 29 and her cumulative GPA was just under 3.3; she applied to 10 medical schools and was accepted to 5.

Dan said that his interest in science had increased "big time" during the past year. He retook the MCAT, after earning a total of 25 on the first attempt. His second score was 30, with all subtests in the double digits, and his cumulative GPA was just under 3.9. He applied to seven schools and was accepted by three. When asked about the negative aspects of the premed experience, he said there were none.

Unlike many of the premeds interviewed, *Lynn* said that her most difficult course was not organic chemistry, but biochemistry. The course was similar to those she would encounter in medical school, the culmination of many science courses. "It was a 'thinking course'; you could not get through on memorizing." Lynn started in premed to make her parents happy, with the knowledge that "I'll be respected, making money, but doing good for the world." Over the past 4 years, she had found her own reasons for staying in medicine and in her senior year was interested in public health, in the United States and abroad. She took the MCAT while studying abroad in her third year, finding the test "very hard." She retook the test in the United States and scored 27. She acknowledged that the premed experience—its academic aspects—was difficult. Yet the experience provided opportunity for personal growth. "I am so appalled at the number of people who want to be doctors but don't know why. The premed process hasn't taught them anything—those who have not seen failure yet, who have not had to question why they are doing it." She applied to seven medical schools and was accepted to one.

Chris took organic chemistry in his third year, earning B+ and B grades in the lecture components of the course. He said that he did well in that course because he spent a great deal of time on it and "could picture the images [chemical structures] very well." He reported that his interest in science had increased during the past year, due primarily to a laboratory-based course in which he had the opportunity to do research. He applied to three medical schools but was not accepted. While his MCAT was 30, a good score, his GPA was only just above 3.00 and his application was late. He planned to reapply. He mentioned as a positive aspect of the premed experience that he had received support from other students. "Some of my best friends are in the premed program. Those who get accepted do not lord it over the rest of us." A negative aspect of the experience was too little advising and too little assistance during the application process. After completing a master's degree, 3 years later, Chris was accepted to medical school.

THESE PROFILES DOCUMENT diversity in this population—their scores were not all in double digits and their grades were not all As. What stands out in the accounts of many of those who would go on to medical school is a sustained interest in and appreciation for the challenge of science, as well as an interest in helping humankind.

Chapter 6

CONCLUSIONS

"I feel prepared for medical school."

"I made a final decision that I am going to call it quits and not look back to regret it. ...I feel bad for those who are still trying to get into medical school by doing what 'looks good' to them."

From the onset, this project was an attempt to understand the factors contributing to a choice to pursue the education for an elite profession. The premeds in this study were more alike than different, when set in the context of the national population of college students. Their high school grades and test scores were above average, some in the superior range. Their families and friends more than likely were supportive of their personal goals, or at least they seldom interfered with progress toward these goals. These premeds were involved in their high schools and in their communities. Consequently, variation in many of the measures used was much reduced, in comparison with what would have been obtained from a larger cross-section of U.S. college students. Yet medical students are not representative of the college student population. And there is variation in these measures of performance, behavior, motivation, support, and demographic and background factors. There were differences between those who persisted in premed and those who did not.

The *process* of preparing for medicine is (or can be) generally known to current and future premed students: Follow a science-intensive curriculum in high school. Devote as much time and effort as necessary to master the content of the high school science and college premed courses. Select some extracurricular activities that focus on health care or at least on serving others. Get experience in a science laboratory, if possible. The obstacle to success is less in any lack of information than in a lack of ability, discipline, or motivation. Yet the outcome of these actions and accomplishments is uncertain, because of an imbalance of supply and demand. Only the best, as defined both quantitatively—with courses taken, grades and MCAT scores earned—and more qualitatively—by the quality of the educational experience, the dedication exhibited in out-of-class activities, and performance in the interview—will be rewarded with the opportunity to advance to higher-level training in medical school.

Adding to the uncertainty is that *best* is defined only in relation to other applicants. There is no specific set of standards that, if met, yields the hoped-for reward of admission. During each undergraduate semester, grades serve as the measure of success, a reason to stay or to leave. The population of nonpersisters becomes more diverse from the first year to the fourth, as students find more reasons to change direction. Some premeds with a low probability of success persist. Others, who might make it, change directions rather than be rejected. Still others find new interests and, in effect, reject medicine. Every student who began in this study had a chance. While some entered college better equipped for the challenge than others, the interview data show that some with weaker high school science and math preparation, including some whose high school chemistry course offered no laboratory component, reached their goal of admission to medical school, some with enormous effort.

REFLECTING ON MEDICINE

This project coincided with proposals on the national level to reform health care in the United States. Extensive public discussion ensued on the accessibility and affordability of health care. An assumption on which this study rested was the attractiveness of medicine as a profession, in part because it was the highest paid and most highly respected of professions, as well as one that produced great social goods. Indeed, the *Statistical Abstract* of 1991 listed physician as one of the occupations in which "largest job growth" was anticipated between 1988 and 2000 (p. 398). But with institutional change likely, although perhaps not as revolutionary as some of the study participants feared in 1993 and 1994, it appears that the highest salaries will decrease—by how much no one knows. And the autonomy of the individual physician has been significantly reduced. The solo practitioner has become rarer still.

The awareness of ongoing or impending change to the medical profession began for some of the premeds in courses on health care policy, medical ethics, or the sociology of medicine. While all premeds were well acquainted with the biological and physical sciences, some of them were having classroom discussions for the first time about the challenges currently facing medicine. How do we as a society make high-quality health care widely available while keeping it affordable? If some rationing is inevitable, on what basis should it be done? Many of the premeds were concerned about these issues, wondering if they were preparing themselves for a profession they would indeed want to be part of later on. The answer to that question was not clear for many of them.

As individuals evaluated their career decision, some came to question their ability, even 2 years into a premed program: "I have a lot of doubt. There are a lot of years involved; I don't know whether I'll make it in medical school and I have nothing to fall back on." Others questioned their dedication: "I'm leaning toward law now; I don't think I have the dedication for medicine. . . . Medicine is not as rewarding as it was in the past, because of malpractice and government regulation." Still others questioned what they wanted in a career: "When I first started, I felt I'd make a lot of money and be a great big name in medicine. Now I see that I won't make as much money [as I had expected to]." Yet some pursued a career in medicine in spite of what they perceived to be some unwelcome changes: "I never wanted general practice, but that looks like what we will have to do to get jobs."

Some premeds came to understand more clearly that the doctor practicing medicine is imbedded in a network of institutional arrangements that an individual practitioner, certainly a newcomer to the profession, is unlikely to change:

> I'm a little worried and scared. . . . Doctors are getting more restricted, seeing more patients, especially in HMOs. Doctors don't want to struggle financially. I don't want to see the government control medicine.

> I had wanted to study medicine to help people. Now I know that it is more of a bureaucracy. Many people can't be helped because they have no insurance.

> Medicine has become so impersonal; doctors don't know your name. People want attention from the doctor and are not getting it. . . . Doctors need to be more compassionate [but instead] have a lot of animosity after going through hell in medical school.

When premed students enter college, they tend to be focused on medicine as a way of doing good for others. During the undergraduate years, many of them begin to see some of the downside of medicine:

> Malpractice insurance is high, doctors' salaries are going down, and the risk of infectious disease is too great.

> The whole AIDS crisis, hepatitis, how communicable diseases can be carried home to my family. [But, she went on to say,] everyone should have access to health care.

By the third year, a small number of premeds had gravitated toward alternative forms of medicine:

> I am interested in exercise physiology and naturopathic medicine. There are two naturopathic medical schools in the U.S., [where] the focus is on health rather than on disease.

> I am now looking at schools of osteopathy. [They] look beyond just grades and MCAT in deciding on admission. They take a more holistic view. Being an MD or a DO is now of no difference to me.

The latter student was not alone in minimizing the distinction between these two approaches to medicine. Many premeds, confronted with the odds against admission to an allopathic school, looked for alternatives, which became more acceptable as the probability of admission to them increased. Admission to schools of osteopathic medicine has become more competitive, too, however, as the perceived distinctions between the two types of practice have further blurred.

The prospect of macro-level change in the funding and delivery of health care means that these premed students cannot learn about their own futures as practicing physicians by observing and talking with older physicians. Lacking the ability to predict the future contributed to any insecurity they already had. Medicine has become more similar to the myriad of occupations that have been transformed by technology, economics, and demographics. If the technology is available, hospitals, doctors, and patients will want it. But there are high costs of keeping up with technology and for the training required to make use of it. Some rationing of care ensues, under the rubric of *managed care*. Emerging technology also contributes to institutional competition in offering *state-of-the art* services. Increased scrutiny is given to patients' requests for specialized medical care and to their general practice physicians who refer them for treatment by specialists. And the population is living longer, with more individuals needing medical care over a longer lifetime. A change in the national employment profile, from manufacturing to services, has changed the income distribution, too. A decreasing percentage of the labor force has secure employment, and a significant percentage of the working population is without health insurance. Those individuals and families without company-provided insurance are not likely to be able to pay for medical care out of their own pockets. Yet the demand for medical care continues to increase.

Awareness among premeds of these macro-level issues was demonstrated during the second and third interviews, in response to a question about changes in their views on medicine and health care. Their answers provided

insight into their personal values and reasons for persisting or not in premed:

> My views are more conservative now. I was in favor of socialized medicine, but not
> now. I worked for a city ambulance service and went into the [public housing] proj-
> ects. I saw exploitation of welfare, also drugs. I felt sorry for a while but now I am
> fed up. (a persister through time 2)

> I went into medicine without thinking of these [macro-level] issues. Now insurance
> companies drive me crazy. They aren't fair to people. Now I am aware that privi-
> leged people have greater access to care. I never thought about giving service away
> to help people. Now I think of this. I may do some of it myself. (a persister through
> time 3)

> I'm scared of where medicine is going. I don't like the way we are leaning toward so-
> cialized medicine. Doctors are moving from a most respected position to one of less
> respect. (a persister through time 2)

> I see more problems with the system [now]; not everyone gets the care they de-
> serve.

> I used to see it naively, as everyone receiving health care. Now I view medicine dif-
> ferently. Perhaps socialized medicine is not a bad thing. (a persister through time 3)

Two years later, this same student was more ambivalent:

> I have found myself feeling more dichotomous. I used to think *liberally*—health care
> for all. Take away from the haves and give to the have-nots. Now I am more con-
> cerned with the quality of care and research. [But] I still favor a national system of
> health care.

One of this respondent's parents is a physician:

> I've seen it close up; I've seen how nonglamorous it is. I'm concerned with the direc-
> tion that policy makers are trying to send medicine, toward nationalized health care,
> like Canada. While that is distasteful to me, it does not deter me from the practice
> of medicine. I want some autonomy, but I will sacrifice some of it, too. Perceptions
> of the medical profession by the general public concern me—about doctors' salaries
> and rising health care costs. They do not understand give-and-take. They want all
> technology available [to them] but they do not want to pay. Doctors and health
> care personnel need to get back to where things were 30 years ago—more caring
> and compassionate. (a persister through time 3)

> I've been thinking more about the possibility of socialized medicine; overall, I think
> that would be a good thing. (a persister through time 3)

> I don't care if we have socialized medicine or not. You don't need so much money. ...There needs to be an overhaul of the health care system [to focus on] insurance companies and high costs. (a persister through time 3)

During the last interview, the subject of rewards came up often, usually in the context of rewards compared with costs or in a discussion of medicine competing for rewards in the new managed-care environment.

AFTER COLLEGE

While this study ended with the acceptance of many of the persisters into one or more medical schools, some of the participants provided some follow-up reports when they were 2 or 3 years out of college:

> Medical school is extremely difficult—harder than any class I have ever taken. It makes [undergraduate classes] seem like a joke.... The practices that supported high performance in college became useless. (Michael)

> When we last spoke in my senior year...I recall that I was still on the waiting lists of three schools....I was finally granted an acceptance in mid-June [for the class starting in August]....Since then, I have been...studying around the clock. (Lynn)

Marsha, in an MD/PhD program, wrote:

> My first 2 years of medical school are completed now. I found the first year basic science classes interesting, but primarily a test of memorization. The second year classes were far more challenging, especially pathology....My performance exceeded my expectations. [Referring to her undergraduate major in psychology]: My work in the lab was a great influence on my decision to pursue a dual MD/PhD degree.

Once in medical school, the competition intensifies, as the best among the highly qualified applicants now compete directly with one another. Even those individuals who earned As in premed science courses occasionally find themselves performing below the satisfactory level in a medical school course. Passing a difficult course can become a source of personal pride. A women who was doing well in a DO program provided some insight into the day-to-day experience of a first year medical student:

> I try my best to understand [the course material], but because of the huge quantity of information and the continuous heavy load, sometimes I find myself memorizing. I always get burned in the end for just memorizing, though, because everything you learn in class is integrated. What you did last month in biochemistry is very likely go-

ing to come up next week in physiology.... I have found that learning to understand allows you to retain much longer. I have also found that to be true of information that I learned [as an undergraduate]. Group studying has been my lifesaver. I believe it is very important because of the huge amounts of information.... It is also very important because it is the only social outlet that I have. You are in class, studying, eating, or sleeping for 23 hours of the day.

Many of the men and women who began college as premed found satisfaction in health care and science-based careers outside medicine. Emily enrolled in a master's program in public health and retook the MCAT, but she said that her heart was no longer in it. She is happy with her career in public health, acknowledging: "I have never been so focused and confident about my career until now." Another premed persister completed a master's degree in public health and enrolled in a doctoral program in that field. One woman persister completed a master's program in microbiology and was employed in medical research:

When I began [college], I had every intention of going to medical school, but two things happened. I became more interested in the science behind medicine and worried that if I did choose to go to med school, then that would be my life. [About her current field]: I feel as though I've made the right choice.

Others made bigger shifts in direction, selecting law, business, or education, to name a few examples. One former premed who persisted through the second year combined his early interest in medicine with his new interest in law. He was in law school, intending to concentrate his legal work in medical malpractice. Another former premed changed direction early: "[I] left any aspiration for medical study in the chemistry lab, at the end of my first year." He joined the Peace Corps, where his experience was "magnificent," and then began a graduate program in a field outside the health sciences.

Just as it was not possible to portray in any detail a *premed type*, the variation in former premeds is even wider. Their immediate options after college depend to a large degree on their most recent performances and accomplishments, inside and outside the classroom. Leaving premed carries no stigma. The program is demanding in many ways and is not for everyone. Staying too long without succeeding, however, does cut off some other attractive options in the immediate future.

THEORY REVISITED

Theory and research on rational behavior, social comparison, and socialization, especially gender socialization, have provided some framework for understanding the premed process. Persons embarking on preparation for medicine try to act as if the process of accumulating credentials and accomplishments while competing with others holding similar ambitions is one that can be understood and whose outcomes can be predicted. For most young adults, the early stages of career preparation are not as ordered as a premed program. There is more than one way to begin a career in business, politics, or teaching, but there is a single path to medical school. It is that fact, and the identifiable sequence of intermediate steps toward the goal, that gives coherence to the decision process. A modified rational decision model could apply to the process of preparing for medicine, especially for the majority of students who selected premed rather than having it selected for them. The model continues to apply for students whose performance is sufficiently high to provide them with choices—between medicine and other professions, and among medical schools. For others, lower or inconsistent performance introduces uncertainty, and the rational model is no longer useful. These students are far less confident of the outcome of their college preparation. Lacking the objective measures of high performance that the highest performers have, they use less reliable measures of achievement, such as social comparisons, while trying to determine how good is *good enough*.

To attempt an answer to that question—will persistence in premed pay off?—premeds will need to know something about students admitted to medical school in the previous year, especially about those who had lower grades or MCAT scores than the average of those who were admitted. They will seek information about unusual extracurricular activities or mitigating factors, and they will try to learn which schools place less weight on grades and scores. In making social comparisons, a student's aim is to find individuals who were accepted to a medical school with a record at that time that was no better than his or hers is now. Since this information is not readily available and must come from the accepted medical student or a close friend of that student, it is often difficult for this year's applicant to make a thorough comparison. If some relevant information is available, even if incomplete, that permits a student to make a favorable comparison with someone already admitted, this will increase confidence and the likelihood of persisting. The experience of taking premed science classes with normative-based grading has illustrated the importance of social comparison. Applicants who do not compare favorably with last year's accepted students may hope for a better comparison group this year—but with recent application-to-acceptance ratios, this is not realistic for most of them.

While imposing rationality on the process may reduce anxiety for the participants, they must attend, too, to the context in which career preparation is taking place, factors that contribute a nonrational element to the process. There is the immediate personal context—the relationship that ended just before a major exam, the loss of a notebook, the loud roommate who keeps late hours. There is the university context—the high caliber of fellow students, the professor judged to be more difficult and less approachable than his or her colleagues in the department, who is teaching this premed course for the first time in years, and the only open lab sections those that are scheduled at hours too early or late to be desirable. And there is the national context—the intense competition for places in the next medical school class, coupled with the national conversation on health care reform, a conversation that still is open-ended. These contexts provide uncertainty at each decision point.

Gender did not emerge as a particularly salient and independent factor for the premed students. The women in this study were as well or better prepared in math and science, on average, than the men. They did not report any systematic gender bias in the premed program, nor did they say they anticipated any in the admission process. Yet, using Fiorentine and Cole's (1992) terminology, while structural barriers have been lowered, normative constraints remain, as women more than men wrestle with the competing desires for a professional career and a family life in which they will participate actively. A difference in performance in favor of men in the study was noted in MCAT scores, but even there, the overlap of women's and men's scores was extensive. At the lower end of the distribution the difference was more pronounced, with more women than men earning scores too low to attract the favorable notice of a medical school.

At the institutional level, conflict theorists have focused attention on the competition of occupations for the rewards available in the society, including income and prestige. Since medicine became the science-based profession with rigorous preparation that it is today, the profession has not had much competition for rewards, or at least has emerged the victor of any such competition. Today that situation is changing for medicine. One characteristic of a profession is self-regulation. The medical profession retains control over licensing and other professional aspects of medicine but has lost some control over financial aspects. Government and insurance companies are participating in and even making decisions that once were solely in the purview of doctors. This regulation from outside the profession has impacted on the freedom of doctors individually and collectively to set the conditions of their practice.

While the conflict perspective is concerned with conflict and control, the functionalist perspective considers the value of the service provided by doctors, the length and cost of their required professional training, and the scarcity of available talent to determine the appropriate level of rewards for practitioners. Today, while doctors perform a highly valued service, perhaps the most highly valued, they are less autonomous individually and less accessible to their patients, who are now more aware of a health care *industry*, where services are performed by specialists, many of whom are not doctors. Fewer Americans today have personal relationships with their doctor, if many of us can be said to *have a doctor* at all, in an HMO setting. There are far more applicants now who are qualified for medical training than can be accommodated. This raises the question for public discussion: Do doctors need to earn so much, especially when the income of so many adults in the population is flat or on the decline? The shift is from *they deserve so much* to *what can we afford to pay*, where *we* are not individual patients but the society as a whole.

SOME STRATEGIES FOR SUCCESS FOR PREMEDS AND PRE-PREMEDS

At the beginning of the book readers were cautioned against expecting a *how-to* book for gaining acceptance to medical school. Yet there are some lessons to be learned from the participants in this study. While advice is plentiful on what to do to succeed in the premed program, it is impossible to know that any particular decision—to take a course, to take the honors section, to join a study group, or to join an emergency medical team—will have the desired outcome. Yet while the outcome for any particular individual will not be known in advance, there are some strategies to improve the *probability* of success. Behaviors and performances contributing to success at different stages, from pre-college to medical school application, will be described, using themes discussed throughout the book: academic performance and supporting behaviors, motivation for medicine, social support and competition, and gender.

High School

A high school student who hopes someday to be a physician should take a full college preparatory science and mathematics curriculum. This course of study should include at least 1 year each of biology, chemistry, and physics, as well as mathematics through the precalculus or calculus level. Many high schools offer a second year of biology, and a smaller number also offer additional chemistry and physics. A future premed student can benefit in more than one way by taking these additional courses. Of most direct benefit is any overlap in course content, usually between the second high school course in the subject and the first college course. A person who completes additional science courses while in high school will become more comfortable with the subject matter—learning how to frame questions and answers, and learning to manipulate new types of information in new ways. A strong background in the subject will enable the student to focus more on understanding the subject in college, rather than just memorizing content. Courses that require investigation and problem solving will be more useful than those that are more descriptive. The contrast is between courses in which students *do* science and those in which they learn *about* science. Successful students are engaged, asking questions in class or afterwards when they do not understand. They can get ahead by reading and practicing math and science outside the classroom, reading books and magazine articles with a science focus, playing challenging games, solving puzzles, learning and modifying or even designing computer applications.

Developing a habit of commitment, focusing on long-term goals while also accumulating short-term achievements, is rewarding later on. The discipline required to progress toward a distant goal while overcoming obstacles en route will be useful in premed and in medical school. Advanced courses in a rigorous curriculum will necessitate reading material twice or more, as well as working on problems until reaching a solution. To find the time necessary to devote to such courses, students can ask for household responsibilities that can be grouped together in blocks of time, freeing up other blocks for study. They can limit the hours of employment unless the job is truly necessary. Selecting a small number of extracurricular activities and staying with them over time can develop personal talents and leadership ability. Leadership is not limited to holding office in an organization but can involve a major role in a dramatic production, a position in a youth orchestra, or organizing a food drive for a community food bank. Persisting in a few activities permits an individual to develop long-term perspective and reap the success that comes from effort expended over time. In any long-term endeavor there will be setbacks. Getting beyond the setbacks or moving in a more self-fulfilling direction can be good practice for the college years and beyond.

Social support is rewarding for those who have it, but its absence need not be defeating. Without abandoning all old friends, prospective premeds should also associate with peers who set serious goals for themselves. They should seek out a teacher or counselor who can provide support for taking a demanding curriculum, especially if there is little support for this at home. While some people think they can go it alone, it can be a great help to have someone to provide encouragement through the difficult times. And one of those difficult times may come in the future—if the goal of entering medical school is not attainable.

All these suggestions—academics through support—are made without regard for the student's gender. The participants in this study have shown that women and men can excel in math and science. Women who are not now hearing this message must find friends and supporters who believe it. They can investigate career programs in school, where they can shadow a professional woman for a day, or volunteer in a setting where there will be contact with women who are physicians or other health care professionals. Sharing aspirations with them and receiving feedback and reinforcement can create a new support group for the prospective premed.

Premed

Once in college, premeds should take their studies seriously, from day one, making academic success their primary goal, *doing the problems at the end of the chapters*. Research has documented that the number of credits completed in undergraduate chemistry correlated positively with MCAT scores; the more chemistry courses, the higher the MCAT (M. L. Hall & Stocks, 1995).

Successful premeds seek out professors, teaching assistants, and tutors when they need minor clarification or are hopelessly lost. Those who continue to be lost as the semester progresses, however, should take this as a sign that this curriculum is not playing to their strengths. Getting advice from the college's premed adviser or another knowledgeable person is recommended. Studying to understand, while recognizing that sometimes it is necessary to memorize some of the content, is preferable to memorizing as the primary study strategy. Some men and women never had to study before entering college and could benefit from short courses on studying, note-taking, and exam preparation if their colleges offer them. Doing the course reading before each class, in a setting without major distraction, helps students to become active listeners in class, which is preferable to attempting to record the professor's lecture in a notebook word-for-word. This study offers no single answer to the question of whether to join study groups or not; half of the participants did and half did not. Working in such groups, even infrequently, can increase participants' comfort level with the material as they learn new perspectives on the issues under discussion and alternative ways of solving problems. Science and medicine outside the classroom are not solo activities. Yet individual students also need to be able to grasp the material well enough to perform on tests. Being able to apply information already learned to new situations gives students ownership of the material and should improve their test performance.

There is some evidence that persons who selected medicine because of its financial rewards are likely to stay in premed longer, even when they are not succeeding. These individuals need to keep in mind that their attraction to the extrinsic rewards of the profession will not improve the probability of admission. For premeds generally, regardless of the specific attraction to medicine, the most difficult advice to take is to consider options other than medical school. It is better to have options and not need them than to finish college with no other plan for the future. The ultimate decision to accept or reject an applicant will be made by each medical school, after comparing his or her performance with those of other qualified applicants. Focusing too much on the magnitude of the competition can be self-defeating, too. To succeed in a premed program, an individual must recognize that it is likely to require a lot of effort. Although a few of the other premeds in the class will not find the courses to be especially difficult; most of them will be working hard, too.

Applying to Medical School

Before beginning the last phase of the premed program, the application stage, premeds should conduct their own research on medical schools. Application fees are high, and prospective medical students will want to target their applications to those schools where they have *any* chance of admission. While it should go without saying that individual should prepare themselves adequately before taking the MCAT, some individual test-takers perform poorly because they have not studied enough or taken practice tests. Performing poorly will reduce or eliminate the possibility of admission that year. Research has shown that the highest correlations with performance in the first year of medical school were with MCAT scores and with undergraduate science GPA (M. L. Hall & Stocks, 1995). A poor performance will delay admission at least a year, if the applicant is still interested. An additional reason to prepare adequately is that some schools will average the scores from the multiple test dates. Skimping on preparation can have permanent consequences.

Before interviewing at a medical school, premeds at college or universities that offer a practice interview should take advantage of that opportunity. A general way to prepare is to anticipate some questions or topics that may be included in an interview. Premeds a year or two ahead can share specific information about interview questions. A likely sort of question concerns recent changes and ongoing trends in health care delivery. The applicant should have thought about some consequences of these changes. Premeds should be able to articulate why they want to be physicians and be able to discuss the positive and negative aspects of their premed experience. What courses, professors, or other persons have been most influential and why? Interviewers may ask applicants to evaluate their strengths and weaknesses. Individuals who tend to get nervous should practice some relaxing techniques so that they can be articulate in the interview setting. Applicants should be acquainted with particular programs, options, and courses at schools where they will interview. If an individual fails to show interest in the interview, the school is likely to look elsewhere to fill its class.

Competition, generally viewed by premeds as negative, can work in their favor. Each medical school wants to fill its next class but not overfill it. Even the stellar applicants can attend only one school, although they, too, may apply to many. No school wants to choose too many applicants who may in turn select another school. The challenge for the medical school is to identify qualified applicants who are *sincerely* interested in attending that school, because of the curriculum, faculty, or opportunities provided, or because the individual hopes to practice medicine in that city or state someday. The choice process, although visible to the individual premed as one-sided, with the schools selecting the next class, is instead a matching process, where both parties are choosing. Medical schools now have a strong advantage, with three times as many applicants as spaces to fill. But this ratio has changed over a relatively short time—and can change again. Recommendations have been made by groups such as the Pew Health Professions Commission to reduce the number of U.S. medical schools (Ginzberg, 1996), which would result in even greater competition. Whatever the specific ratio in a given year, however, there is no evidence that the factors that contributed to the success of the men and women described here are about to change.

REFERENCES

Association of American Medical Colleges (AAMC). (1989). Matriculating student questionnaire. SAIMS database, Washington.

Association of American Medical Colleges (AAMC). (1994a). Characteristics of MCAT examinees 1992–1993. Washington, DC: Author.

Association of American Medical Colleges (AAMC). (1994b). Facts: Applicants, matriculants and graduates. Washington, DC: Author.

Association of American Medical Colleges (AAMC). (1995). Functions and structure of a medical school. Washington, DC: Author.

Altman, L. K. (1993, May 18). Medical schools discover an unexpected popularity. *New York Times*, pp. A1, A10.

Astin, A. (1978). The undergraduate woman. In H. S. Astin & W. Z. Hirsch (Eds.), *The higher education of women* (95–112). New York: Praeger.

Astin, A. W. (1990, January 24). The American freshman: National norms for fall, 1989. *The Chronicle of Higher Education* pp. A33–A34.

Bandura, A. (1977). *Social learning theory.* Englewood Cliffs, NJ: Prentice-Hall.

Bartlett, J. W. (1969). Changes in entering medical students. In R. G. Page & M. H. Littlemeyer (Eds.), *Preparation for the study of medicine* (pp. 129–139). Chicago: University of Chicago Press.

Becker, H. S., Geer, B., Hughes, E. C., & Strauss, A. L. (1961). *Boys in white: Student culture in medical school.* Chicago: University of Chicago Press.

Benbow, C. P., & Stanley, J. C. (1980). Sex differences in mathematical ability: Fact or artifact? *Science, 210,* 1262–1264.

Benbow, C. P., & Stanley, J. C. (1982). Consequences in high school and college of sex differences in mathematical reasoning ability: A longitudinal perspective. *American Educational Research Journal, 19,* 598–622.

Bergquist, S. R., Duchac, B. W., Schalin, V. A., Zastrow, J. F., Barr, V. L., & Borowiecki, T. (1985). Perceptions of freshman medical students of gender differences in medical specialty choice. *Journal of Medical Education, 60,* 379–383.

Berlant, J. L. (1975). *Profession and monopoly.* Berkeley: University of California Press.

Betz, N. E. (1994a). Basic issues and concepts in career counseling for women. In B. Walsh & S. H. Osipow (Eds.), *Career counseling for women* (pp. 1–41). Hillsdale, NJ: Erlbaum.

Betz, N. E. (1994b). Career counseling for women in the sciences and engineering. In W. B. Walsh & S. H. Osipow (Eds.), *Career counseling for women* (pp. 237–261). Hillsdale, NJ: Erlbaum.

Betz, N. E., & Hackett, G. (1981). The relationship of mathematics-related self-efficacy expectations to perceived career options in college women and men. *Journal of Counseling Psychology, 28*, 329–345.

Beutel, A. M., & Marini, M. M. (1995). Gender and values. *American Sociological Review, 60*, 436–448.

Birns, B., & Sternglanz, S. H. (1983). Sex-role socialization: Looking back and looking ahead. In M. B. Liss (Ed.), *Social and cognitive skills* (pp. 235–251). New York: Academic Press.

Bloom, S. W. (1973). *Power and dissent in the medical school.* New York: Free Press.

Boli, J., Allen, M. L., & Payne, A. (1985). High ability women and men in undergraduate mathematics and chemistry courses. *American Educational Research Journal, 22*, 605–626.

Bose, C. E. (1985). *Jobs and gender: A study of occupational prestige.* New York: Praeger.

Bullough, V. L. (1966). *The development of medicine as a profession.* New York: Hafner.

Burke, P. J. (1989). Gender identity, sex, and school performance. *Social Psychology Quarterly, 52*, 159–169.

Burkham, D. T., Lee, V. E., Smerdon, B. A. (1997). Gender and science learning in high school: Subject matter and laboratory experiences. *American Educational Research Journal, 34*, 297–331.

Cage, M. C. (1994, January 26). Beyond the B. A. *The Chronicle of Higher Education,* pp. A21–A31.

Canaday, S. D., & Lancaster, C. J. (1985). Impact of undergraduate courses on medical student performance in basic sciences. *Journal of Medical Education, 60*, 757–762.

Carney, M., & Morgan, C. S. (1981). Female college persisters: Nontraditional versus traditional career fields. *Journal of College Student Personnel, 22*, 418–423.

Cartwright, L. K. (1972). Conscious factors entering into decisions of women to study medicine. *Journal of Social Issues, 28*, 201–215.

Casserly, P. L. (1980). Factors affecting female participation in advanced placement programs in mathematics, chemistry, and physics. In L. H. Fox, L. Brody, & D. Tobin (Eds.), *Women and the mathematical mystique* (pp. 138–163). Baltimore: Johns Hopkins University Press.

Clapp, T., & Reid, J. (1976). Institutional selectivity as a predictor of applicant selection and success in medical school. *Journal of Medical Education, 51*, 850–852.

Cole, S. (1986). Sex discrimination and admission to medical school, 1929–1984. *American Journal of Sociology, 92*, 549–567.

College of Arts and Sciences announcement for 1932–33. (1932). *Bulletin of Tulane University, 33*. New Orleans: Tulane University Press.

Colquitt, W. L., & Killian, C. D. (1991). Students who consider medicine but decide against it. *Academic Medicine, 66,* 273–278.

Connor, J. M., Schackman, M. E., & Serbin, L. A. (1978). Sex-related differences in response to practice on a visual-spatial test and generalization to a related test. *Child Development, 49,* 24–29.

Corder, B. W. (Ed.). (1994). *Medical professions admission guide* (3rd ed.). Champaign, IL: National Association of Advisors for the Health Professions.

Coser, L. A. (1974). *Greedy institutions.* New York: Free Press.

Dahrendorf, R. (1959). *Class and class conflict in industrial society.* Stanford, CA: Stanford University Press.

Davis, J. A. (1967). The campus as frog pond. *American Journal of Sociology, 72,* 17–31.

Davis, K., & Moore, W. E. (1945). Some principles of stratification. *American Sociological Review, 10,* 242–249.

Deaux, K. (1984). From individual differences to social categories. *American Psychologist, 39,* 105–116.

DeBoer, G. E. (1984). A study of gender effects in the science and mathematics course-taking behavior of a group of students who graduated from college in the late 1970s. *Journal of Research in Science Teaching, 21,* 95–103.

Drew, D. E., & Astin, A. W. (1972). Undergraduate aspirations: A test of several theories. *American Journal of Sociology, 77,* 1151–1164.

Eccles, J. (1994). Understanding women's educational and occupational choices. *Psychology of Women Quarterly, 18,* 585–609.

Eccles, J. S., & Jacobs, J. E. (1986). Social forces shape math attitudes and performance. *Signs, 11,* 367–380.

Eckholm, E. (1993, November 7). Health plan is toughest on doctors making most. *New York Times,* pp. 1, 13.

Elam, C. L., & Johnson, M. S. (1997a). The effect of a rolling admission policy on a medical school's selection of applicants. *Academic Medicine, 72,* 644–646.

Elam, C. L., & Johnson, M. S. (1997b). An analysis of admission committee voting patterns. *Academic Medicine, 72,* S72–S75.

Entwisle, D. R., Alexander, K. L., & Olson, L. S. (1994). The gender gap in math: Possible origins in neighborhood effects. *American Sociological Review, 59,* 822–838.

Etzioni, A. (1992). Normative-affective factors: Toward a new decision-making model. In M. Zey (Ed.), *Decision making* (pp. 89–111). Newbury Park, CA: Sage.

Fennema, E. (1980). Sex-related differences in mathematics achievement: Where and why. In L. H. Fox, L. Brody, & D. Tobin (Eds.), *Women and the mathematical mystique* (pp. 76–93). Baltimore: Johns Hopkins University Press.

Fennema, E. (1984). Girls, women, and mathematics. In E. Fennema & M. J. Ayer (Eds.), *Women and education* (pp. 137–164). Berkeley: McCutchan.

Fennema, E., & Ayer, M. J. (Eds.). (1984). *Women and education.* Berkeley: McCutchan.

Fennema, E., & Peterson, P. (1985). Autonomous learning behavior: A possible explanation of gender-related differences in mathematics. In L. C. Wilkinson & C. B. Marrett (Eds.), *Gender influences and classroom interaction* (pp. 17–35). New York: Academic Press.

Fennema, E., & Sherman, J. A. (1977). Sex-related differences in mathematics achievement, spatial visualization and affective factors. *American Educational Research Journal, 14*, 51–71.

Festinger, L. (1954). A theory of social comparison processes. *Human Relations, 7*, 117–140.

Fiorentine, R. (1988a). Increasing similarities in the values and life plans of male and female college students? Evidence and implications. *Sex Roles, 18*, 143–158.

Fiorentine, R. (1988b). Sex differences in success expectancies and causal attributions: Is this why fewer women become physicians? *Social Psychology Quarterly, 51*, 236–249.

Fiorentine, R., & Cole, S. (1992). Why fewer women become physicians: Explaining the premed persistence gap. *Sociological Forum, 7*, 469–496.

Flexner, A. (1910). *Medical education in the United States and Canada.* New York: Carnegie Foundation for the Advancement of Teaching.

Folger, J. K., & Nam, C. B. (1967). *Education of the American population.* Washington, DC: U.S. Department of Commerce, Bureau of the Census.

Fox, L. (1974). *Facilitating the development of mathematical talent in young women.* Unpublished doctoral dissertation, Johns Hopkins University, Baltimore, MD.

Freidson, E. (1970). *Professional dominance: The social structure of medical care.* Chicago: Aldine.

Friedman, L. (1995). The space factor in mathematics: Gender differences. *Review of Educational Research, 65*, 22–50.

Friedman, M. (1962). *Capitalism and freedom.* Chicago: University of Chicago Press.

Funkenstein, D. H. (1978). *Medical students, medical schools and society during five eras: Factors affecting the career choices of physicians 1958–76.* Cambridge, MA: Ballinger.

Ginsberg, E., Ginsberg, S. W., Axelrod, S., & Herma, J. L. (1951). *Occupational choice: An approach to general theory.* New York: Columbia University Press.

Ginzberg, E. (1996). The future supply of physicians. *Academic Medicine, 71*, 1147–1153.

Goldstein, B., & Oldham, J. (1979). *Children and work: A study of socialization.* New Brunswick, NJ: Transaction.

Gose, B. (1995a, November 24). Panel calls for major cuts in medical-school enrollment. *The Chronicle of Higher Education*, p. A30.

Gose, B. (1995b, November 3). Women's place in medicine. *The Chronicle of Higher Education*, pp. A49–A50.

Gruder, C. (1977). Choice of comparison persons in evaluating oneself. In J. Suls & R. Miller (Eds.), *Social comparison processes* (pp. 21–41). Washington, DC: Halstead.

H. Sophie Newcomb Memorial College for Women announcement for 1920–21. (1920). *Bulletin of Tulane University, 21*. New Orleans: Tulane University Press.

H. Sophie Newcomb Memorial College for Women announcement for 1932–33. (1932). *Bulletin of Tulane University, 33*. New Orleans: Tulane University Press.

Hackman, J. D., Low-Beer, J. R., Wugmeister, S., Wilhelm, R. C., & Rosenbaum, J. E. (1979). The premed stereotype. *Journal of Medical Education, 4*, 308–313.

Hall, F. R., & Bailey, B. A. (1992). Correlating students' undergraduate science GPA's, their MCAT scores, and the academic caliber of their undergraduate colleges with their first-year academic performances across five classes at Dartmouth Medical School. *The Advisor, 12*, 3–6.

Hall, M. L., & Stocks, M. T. (1995). Relationship between quantity of undergraduate science preparation and preclinical performance in medical school. *Academic Medicine, 70*, 230–235.

Handel, R. D. (1986, April, 16–20). *Achievement attitudes in mathematics and science: Relationships between self-perceptions, aspirations, and extracurricular activities.* Paper presented at the meeting of the American Educational Research Association, San Francisco.

Hanson, E. D. (1969). Trends in college biology: Teaching a new life science. In R. G. Page & M. H. Littlemeyer (Eds.), *Preparation for the study of medicine* (pp. 83–95). Chicago: University of Chicago Press.

Harris, L. J. (1979). Sex-related differences in spatial ability: A developmental psychological view. In C. B. Kopp (Ed.), *Becoming female* (pp. 133–181). New York: Plenum.

Hartley, J., & Cameron, J. (1967). Some observations on the efficiency of lecturing. *Educational Review, 20*, 3–7.

Hartley, J., & Marshall, S. (1974). On notes and notetaking. *Universities Quarterly, 28*, 225–235.

Hearn, J. C., & Olzak, S. (1981). The role of college major departments in the reproduction of sexual inequality. *Sociology of Education, 54*, 195–205.

Hedges, L. V., & Nowell, A. (1995). Sex differences in mental test scores, variability, and numbers of high-scoring individuals. *Science, 269*, 41–45.

Hilton, T. L., & Berglund, G. W. (1974). Sex differences in mathematics achievement: A longitudinal study. *Journal of Educational Research, 67*, 231–237.

Holden, C. (1987). Female math anxiety on the wane. *Science, 236*, 660–661.

Howe, M. J. (1970). Using students' notes to examine the role of the individual learner in acquiring meaningful subject matter. *Journal of Educational Research, 64*, 61–63.

Hyman, H. H. (1968). *Readings in reference group theory and research.* New York: Free Press.

Jacobs, J. E. (1991). Influence of gender stereotypes on parent and child mathematics attitudes. *Journal of Educational Psychology, 83*, 518–527.

Johnson, D. G. (1983). *Physicians in the making: Personal, academic, and socioeconomic characteristics of medical students from 1950 to 2000.* San Francisco: Jossey-Bass.

Johnson, E. K., & Edwards, J. C. (1991). Current practices in admission interviews at U.S. medical schools. *Academic Medicine, 66*, 408–412.

Jones, R., & Adams, L. (1983). The relationship between MCAT science scores and undergraduate science GPA. *Journal of Medical Education, 58*, 908–911.

Kahle, J. B., & Lakes, M. K. (1983). The myth of equality in science classrooms. *Journal of Research in Science Teaching, 20*, 131–140.

Kassebaum, D. G., & Szenas, P. L. (1995). The decline and rise of the medical school applicant pool. *Academic Medicine, 70,* 334–340.

Katchadourian, H. A., & Boli, J. (1994). *Cream of the crop.* New York: Basic Books.

Kelly, A. (Ed.). (1987). *Science for girls.* Milton Keynes, UK: Open University Press.

Kerr, B., & Maresh, S. E. (1994). Career counseling for gifted women. In W. Walsh, W. Bruce, & S. H. Osipow (Eds.), *Career counseling for women* (pp. 197–235). Hillsdale, NJ: Erlbaum.

King, A. (1992). Comparison of self-questioning, summarizing, and notetaking-review as strategies for learning from lectures. *American Educational Research Journal, 29,* 303–323.

Kutner, N. G., & Brogan, D. R. (1980). The decision to enter medicine: Motivations, social support, and discouragements for women. *Psychology of Women Quarterly, 5,* 341–358.

Lemkau, J. P. (1979). Personality and background characteristics of women in male-dominated occupations: A review. *Psychology of Women Quarterly, 4,* 221–240.

Leserman, J. (1981). *Men and women in medical school.* New York: Praeger.

Lewis, G. L. (1984). Academic origins of medical school applicants and entrants 1980–82. *Journal of Medical Education, 59,* 825–828.

Liaison Committee on Medical Education. (1995). *Functions and structure of a medical school.* Washington, DC: Author.

Linn, M. C., & Peterson, A. C. (1985). Emergence and characterization of sex differences in spatial ability: A meta-analysis. *Child Development, 56,* 1479–1498.

Lopate, C. (1968). *Women in medicine.* Baltimore, MD: Johns Hopkins University Press.

Ludmerer, K. M. (1983). *Learning to heal: The development of American medical education.* New York: Basic Books.

Maccoby, E. E., & Jacklin, C. N. (1974). *Psychology of sex differences.* Palo Alto, CA: Stanford University Press.

MacKay, W. R., & Miller, C. A. (1982). Relations of SES and sex variables to the complexity of worker functions in the occupational choices of elementary school children. *Journal of Vocational Behavior, 20,* 31–37.

Mandelbaum, D. (1981). *Work, marriage, and motherhood: The career persistence of women physicians.* New York: Praeger.

Manning, W. D. (1990). Parenting employed teenagers. *Youth and Society, 22,* 184–200.

March, J. G. (1994). *A primer on decision making.* New York: Free Press.

Marini, M. M., & Greenberger, E. (1978). Sex differences in occupational aspirations and expectations. *Sociology of Work and Occupations, 5,* 147–177.

Marsh, H. W. (1991). Employment during high school: Character building or a subversion of academic goals? *Sociology of Education, 64,* 172–189.

McGaghie, W. C. (1990). Perspectives on medical school admission. *Academic Medicine, 65,* 136–139.

McLure, G. T., & Piel, E. (1978). College-bound girls and science careers: Perceptions of barriers and facilitating factors. *Journal of Vocational Behavior, 12,* 172–183.

Medical school admission requirements 1992–93 (42nd ed.). (1991). Washington, DC: Association of American Medical Colleges.

Meece, J. L., Parsons, J. E., Kaczala, C. M., Goff, S. B., & Futterman, R. (1982). Sex differences in math achievement: Toward a model of academic choice. *Psychological Bulletin, 91,* 324–348.

Merton, R. K., Reader, G. G., & Kendall, P. L. (Eds.). (1957). *The student physician.* Cambridge, MA: Harvard University Press.

Meyer, J. W. (1972). The effects of the institutionalization of colleges in society. In K. A. Feldman (Ed.), *College and student* (pp. 109–126). New York: Pergamon.

Michaels, J. W., & Miethe, T. D. (1989). Academic effort and college grades. *Social Forces, 68,* 309–319.

Mitchell, K. J. (1987). Use of MCAT data in selecting students for admission to medical school. *Journal of Medical Education, 62,* 871–879.

Moll, R. W. (1991). *The lure of the law.* New York: Penguin.

Muller, S. (1984). Physicians for the twenty-first century. *Journal of Medical Education, 59* (Part 2), 1–56.

Nachtreib, N. H. (1969). Changing patterns in undergraduate chemistry. In R. G. Page & M. H. Littlemeyer (Eds.), *Preparation for the study of medicine* (pp. 97–102). Chicago: University of Chicago Press.

Oakes, J. (1990). Opportunities, achievement and choice: Women and minority students in science and mathematics. *Review of Research in Education, 16,* 153–222.

Olmstead, A. L., & Sheffrin, S. M. (1981). The medical school admission process: An empirical investigation. *Journal of Human Resources, 16,* 459–467.

Pallas, A. M., & Alexander, K. L. (1983). Sex differences in quantitative SAT performance: New evidence on the differential coursework hypothesis. *American Educational Research Journal, 20,* 165–182.

Parsons, J. E., Adler, T. F., & Kaczala, C. M. (1982). Socialization of achievement attitudes and beliefs: Parental influences. *Child Development, 53,* 310–331.

Peper, R. J., & Mayer, R. E. (1986). Generative effects of note-taking during science lectures. *Journal of Educational Psychology, 78,* 34–38.

Plantz, S., Lorenzo, N. Y., & Cole, J. A. (1993). *Getting into medical school: Strategies for the 90's* (2nd ed.). New York: Prentice-Hall.

Radius, S. M., Becker, M. H., Smith, R., & Katasky, M. E. (1979). The rejected medical school applicant: Sex differences in attitudes and outcomes. *Journal of the American Medical Women's Association, 34,* 208–210, 215–220.

Ramsbottom-Lucier, M., Johnson, M. M. S., & Elam, C. L. (1995). Age and gender differences in students' preadmission qualifications and medical school performances. *Academic Medicine, 70,* 236–239.

Rayack, E. (1967). *Professional power and American medicine.* Cleveland: World Publishing Company.

Riesman, D. (1980). *On higher education: The academic enterprise in an era of rising student consumerism.* San Francisco: Jossey-Bass.

Robbins, L. S., Fantone, J. C., Oh, M. S., Alexander, G. L., Schlafer, M., & Davis, W. K. (1995). The effect of pass/fail grading on first-year students' performances and satisfaction. *Academic Medicine, 70,* 327–329.

Rosenthal, E. (1994, June 25). Doctors who once spurned H.M.O.'s now often find systems' doors shut. *New York Times* (national edition), p. 9.

Shaw, D. L., Martz, D. M., Lancaster, C. J., & Sade, R. M. (1995). Influence of medical school applicants' demographic and cognitive characteristics on interviewers' ratings of noncognitive traits. *Academic Medicine, 70,* 532–536.

Sherman, J. (1983). Factors predicting girls' and boys' enrollment in college preparatory mathematics. *Psychology of Women Quarterly, 7,* 272–281.

Shryock, R. H. (1928). Selections from the letters of Richard D. Arnold: Medical series, 1834–1875. *Bulletin of the Johns Hopkins Hospital, 42,* 156. Quoted in Shryock, R. H., 1966, *Medicine in America: Historical essays.* Baltimore: Johns Hopkins Press.

Siegel, C. L. F. (1973). Sex differences in the occupational choices of second graders. *Journal of Vocational Behavior, 3,* 15–19.

Simon, H. (1957). *Administrative behavior.* New York: Free Press.

Spade, J. Z., Columba, L., & Vanfossen, B. E. (1997). Tracking in mathematics and science: Courses and course-selection procedures. *Sociology of Education, 70,* 108–127.

Starr, P. (1982). *The social transformation of American medicine.* New York: Basic Books.

Statistical abstract of the United States 1991. (1991). Washington, DC: U.S. Department of Commerce, Bureau of the Census.

Steen, L. A. (1987). Mathematics education: A predictor of scientific competitiveness. *Science, 237,* 251–252, 302.

Steinberg, L., Fegley, S., & Dornbusch, S. M. (1993). Negative impact of part-time work on adolescent adjustment: Evidence from a longitudinal study. *Developmental Psychology, 29,* 171–180.

Steincamp, M. W., & Maehr, M. L. (1984). Gender differences in motivational orientations toward achievement in school science: A quantitative synthesis. *American Educational Research Journal, 21,* 39–59.

Tidball, M. E. (1985). Baccalaureate origins of entrants into American medical schools. *Journal of Higher Education, 56,* 385–402.

Tobias, S. (1990, July/August). They're not dumb; They're different. *Change, 22,* 11–30.

Tracy, D. M. (1987). Toys, spatial ability, and science and mathematics achievement: Are they related? *Sex Roles, 17,* 115–138.

Treisman, U. (1992). Studying students studying calculus: A look at the lives of minority mathematics students in college. *The College Mathematics Journal, 23,* 362–372.

Tudor, C. G., & Beran, R. L. (1987). Changes in the qualifications of medical school applicants, 1981 to 1985. *Journal of Medical Education, 62,* 562–571.

Van der Meij, H. (1988). Constraints on question asking in classrooms. *Journal of Educational Psychology, 80,* 401–405.

Waite, L. J., & Berryman, S. E. (1985). *Women in non-traditional occupations.* Santa Monica, CA: Rand Corporation.

Walsh, W. B., & Osipow, S. H. (Eds.). (1994). *Career counseling for women.* Hillsdale, NJ: Erlbaum.

Ware, N. C., & Lee, V. E. (1988). Sex differences in choice of college science majors. *American Educational Research Journal, 25*, 593–614.

Weick, K. E. (1995). *Sensemaking in organizations.* Thousand Oaks, CA: Sage.

What Americans really think about lawyers. (1986). *The National Law Journal, 8*, S1, S19.

White, L. K., & Brinkerhoff, D. B. (1981a). Children's work in the family: Its significance and meaning. *Journal of Marriage and the Family, 43*, 789–798.

White, L. K., & Brinkerhoff, D. B. (1981b). The sexual division of labor: Evidence from childhood. *Social Forces, 60*, 170–181.

Wilson, R. C., Gass, G. G., Dienst, E. R., Wood, L., & Barry, J. L. (1975). *College professors and their impact on students.* New York: Wiley.

Women increasing in medical schools. (1995, May 31). *New Orleans Times Picayune*, p. A9.

Yee, D. K., & Eccles, J. S. (1988). Parent perceptions and attributions for children's math achievement. *Sex Roles, 19*, 317–333.

Index

Subjects

About the Author

Mary Ann Maguire earned her Ph.D. in Sociology from Stanford University and her B.A. in Sociology from Emmanuel College. Her previous scholarship has focused on work and organizations, and on comparisons of Japanese- and American-owned companies. She was on the faculty of The Catholic University of America and is now Associate Dean for Academic Affairs of H. Sophie Newcomb College of Tulane University.